YOGA *for* CLIMBERS

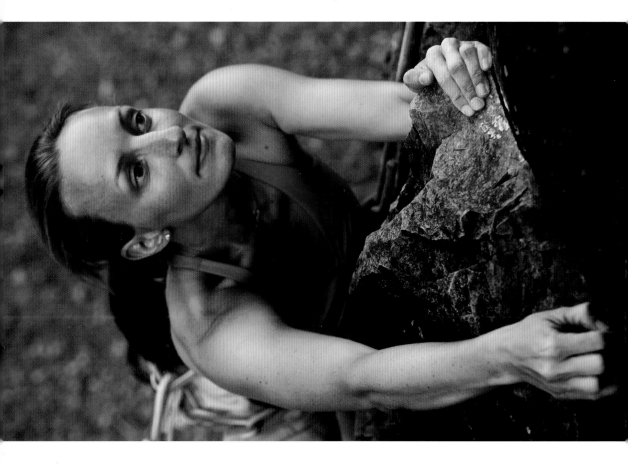

YOGA *for* CLIMBERS

HOW TO STRETCH, STRENGTHEN, *and* CLIMB HIGHER

NICOLE TSONG
PHOTOGRAPHY BY ERIKA SCHULTZ

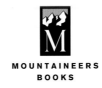

MOUNTAINEERS
BOOKS

TO MY SISTER, INGRID

MOUNTAINEERS BOOKS

Mountaineers Books is the publishing division of The Mountaineers, an organization founded in 1906 and dedicated to the exploration, preservation, and enjoyment of outdoor and wilderness areas.

1001 SW Klickitat Way, Suite 201 • Seattle, WA 98134
800.553.4453 • www.mountaineersbooks.org

Printed in China
Distributed in the United Kingdom by Cordee, www.cordee.co.uk
First edition: first printing 2016, second printing 2019

Copy editor: Nancy Waddell Cortelyou, Saffron Writes
Design: Heidi Smets Graphic Design
Layout: Jennifer Shontz, www.redshoedesign.com
Illustrator: Anna-Lisa Notter, www.annalisanotter.com
Cover photograph: *Bouldering*
Frontispiece: *Focused on the next move*

Library of Congress Cataloging-in-Publication Data
Names: Tsong, Nicole, author. | Schultz, Erika, photographer.
Title: Yoga for climbers : how to stretch, strengthen, and climb higher / Nicole Tsong ; photography by Erika Schultz.
Description: Seattle, WA : Mountaineers Books, [2016] | Includes bibliographical references and index.
Identifiers: LCCN 2015041155 | ISBN 9781594859953 (pbk.)
Subjects: LCSH: Hatha yoga. | Mountaineering. | Endurance sports—Training. | Exercise.
Classification: LCC RC1220.Y64 T75 2016 | DDC 613.7/046—dc23
LC record available at http://lccn.loc.gov/2015041155

Mountaineers Books titles may be purchased for corporate, educational, or other promotional sales, and our authors are available for a wide range of events. For information on special discounts or booking an author, contact our customer service at 800-553-4453 or mbooks@mountaineersbooks.org.

ISBN (paperback): 978-1-59485-995-3
ISBN (ebook): 978-1-59485-996-0

An independent nonprofit publisher since 1960

CONTENTS

ACKNOWLEDGMENTS

WRITING A BOOK IS a tremendous adventure, and there are many people and communities whose generosity of spirit and big love helped me arrive here.

To my parents, Joanna and Peter, thank you for your unwavering love and support. To my sister Ingrid, thank you for your love, early edits, and patient listening.

To my teacher Baron Baptiste, thank you for a methodology that is my teaching source. To the bright light Susanne Conrad, thank you for teaching me to hear and embrace why I am on the planet, and for sharing igolu with the world.

To Michel Spruance, thank you for early rounds of feedback, for modeling, and for your faith in me. To Tina Templeman, thank you for your enthusiasm and support at all levels of the project, from photo shoots to anatomy.

To the models in these pages—Natalie Wieder, Sam Young, Mercedes Pollmeier, Taylor Moravec, G. Webster Ross IV, Tina Templeman, Brian Charlton, Austin Carrillo, Paul Javid, Genevieve Alvarez, and Peter and Michel Spruance—your athleticism, can-do spirit, and playfulness are an inspiration. To Gaylinyet Roberts, thank you for illuminating our inner beauty.

To my Be Luminous Yoga, Shakti Vinyasa Yoga, igolu, Lululemon Pacific Place, and Baptiste communities—thank you for being the best.

To the staff at Mountaineers Books, thank you for your partnership and vision. To the climbers and experts who embraced this book, thank you for contributing your wisdom. To the staff at *Pacific Northwest* magazine at the *Seattle Times*—thank you for "Fit for Life."

To Erika Schultz, thank you for capturing our vision so beautifully.

To my favorite hiking and bouldering partner, Chris, thank you for being hilarious and direct, for holding me to my best self, and for your love.

INTRODUCTION

I STARTED CLIMBING AFTER I started teaching yoga. Despite my best intentions, some days my yoga training flitted away while I was on a wall. The circumstances varied, but those lapses typically involved moments when I was facing a move just beyond my skill level, or my fingers and forearms were screaming. Suddenly, I'd remember *I'm high up*. My heart thudded louder and faster. I reached for chalk for newly sweating palms. I panted a bit and wondered if it was time to call "take" and wait for my belayer to lower me.

Fortunately, feeling panicky didn't last forever. At some point, I remembered to pause. I composed myself: I found a comfortable stance, I loosened my death grip on the holds, and I shook out my arms. I took a deep breath in, exhaled all the way out—and looked again at the problem in front of me. I'd usually notice a tiny hold I'd missed earlier. Or realize if I turned my hips and changed the position of my feet, I could get to the next move.

Or I'd finally hear my belayer calling out a brilliant suggestion from below. Whichever way it went, I'd make my move and climb on.

People often say climbing is like yoga, only higher up. Climbers understand on an intimate level the need to stay focused and present. If they don't, they make mistakes. As a climber, you know the extraordinary mental focus it takes to hang on to a tiny crimp, and with grace and concentration, move through the challenging crux of a tough route. You know the commitment and faith required to tackle—and send—a next-level climb. You've witnessed your own transformation, climbing harder than you ever thought possible, and you've been inspired by others when they have done it too. Focus has taken root in your bones and tissue, with the lessons gained from route after route now embedded in your fingertips and feet.

In yoga, I have questioned my own physical strength—and experienced what it was like to break through. When I first started to practice, I had moved from Anchorage, Alaska, to Seattle. It was summer, and I chose yoga to cope with the new obstacles of traffic and living at a latitude where the sun faded away at 9 p.m. rather than at midnight. I hoped yoga would strengthen my shoulders. I figured I could work on my core, an eternally weak area.

I dove headfirst into a heated power flow practice; I had never sweated so much in my life. I loved feeling my legs burn while holding poses, even as I mentally begged the teacher to let us release out of the pose. I adored the little snooze I snuck in during the final rest at the end of each class. I was sore for days after. Each time, I felt rinsed out, and I had let go of stress from work. I was exhausted in the best way.

Back then, I would give myself a day or two to recover, and return to my mat. One teacher said if your heart rate was up, it was proof you were building cardiovascular strength. Her arms were ripped, and she only did yoga. I wanted to believe her claim. But as much as I loved yoga, I didn't believe it could turn an active twenty-something into an athlete.

That winter, on my first trip to the ski trails outside Seattle, instead of pausing halfway up every hill, I made it all the way to the top. On every single hill. I was panting each time, sure, but I had done it. I was astonished. Until that point, I only knew a world where I had to stop during the first climb of the season, gasping for air to fuel my burning legs. It usually took me at least a month to ski up to about 4 miles (7 kilometers) in one go without pause—and here I was practically bolting up the hills on the first day.

Like climbing, yoga requires both strength and flexibility, and through a regular yoga practice, I gained both. In those early days of yoga, it was a struggle to touch my toes, but now I can hold the bottoms of my feet. I can bear my own body weight and more: My understanding of how my body moves in space has grown exponentially. My endurance for long summer hikes and winter skis expanded, and my recovery time shrank. The experience also made me excited to try new physical activities, from kickboxing and learning to row a single scull, to climbing and bouldering.

I was so excited to learn new poses and so inspired by my new inner athlete that it took time for me to understand that being able to do a pose is not the point of yoga, just as climbing is not ultimately about the difficulty of climbs. Stay with me here. I realized that even if I hadn't grabbed my feet in a Seated Forward Fold, I still emerged feeling light and free. Just as you might tackle a boulder problem for days or even weeks before solving it, and yet you still leave feeling grounded and focused—and determined to work on it again.

Yoga showed me a different path to achieving an experience of freedom and peace that once required an elevation gain of at least 3000 feet on a hike. On a yoga mat in a warm room deep in the heart of a bustling city, I learned to push myself physically, to breathe in a new way, and to feel that same sense of grounding and serenity I feel when hiking up to the clouds.

Yoga showed me what it meant to be present. I have learned that when I am in the moment, I let go of thoughts that tell me I am not strong or flexible enough for a pose. When I experience my body as stronger and more agile than I have known it to be, my idea of my body's boundaries dissolve, and the limitations I have put on myself and my life evaporate. You've felt it when you climb. You have seen when you are committed, focused, and present, your training kicks in. Suddenly, a climb that once felt out of reach is right there in front of you.

A regular yoga practice—by which I mean two to three times a week or more—is a reliable way to enhance your physical strength on the wall, regardless of your condition. Yoga opens your body to new mobility: It balances your strength in your shoulders and core, increases core strength and overall durability for long days of hauling heavy gear, and stretches out tight hips.

Yoga also teaches you to listen to your body on a deeper level, observing the times to push and the times to take your intensity down a notch. Your understanding of how your body moves in space will shift. You may notice you can relax your face instead of gritting your teeth before an intense move. You may have more ease when you rest on the wall. You will find it easier to focus on breath to make tough moves, and to lower your heart rate quickly despite the effort it took to get there.

Breath helps you focus on what you're doing in that moment, and most climbers underestimate the importance of breath, says Christine Deyo, former head setter at the Seattle Bouldering Project.

If you want to be a strong climber and push limits, you have to find that mental focus. "Every climber should do yoga," she says.

Climbers often live to conquer the next route, always seeking the next challenge, the next adventure, the next climb to send. A yoga practice can support all of those goals and surprise you with some additional benefits. You may be startled to understand more deeply why you love challenge and how to stay balanced and unattached in the midst of it all.

YOGA HAS EXPLODED IN popularity since I started practicing more than ten years ago. *Yoga Journal*, the leading national yoga magazine, and Yoga Alliance, a national trade association, recently released a study that showed more than thirty-six million Americans practice yoga. More than eighty million Americans—or thirty-four percent of the population—say they are likely to practice yoga in the next twelve months for reasons including flexibility, stress relief, and fitness. Yoga has emerged from being a trend in the early 2000s to a mainstream activity for active Americans.

Athletes of all types now tout yoga as part of their training. Snowboard slopestyle 2014 Olympic gold medalist Jamie Anderson and basketball superstar LeBron James are among the high-profile athletes who speak about the benefits of a regular yoga practice. The Seattle Seahawks famously meditated on their path to the 2014 Super Bowl championship.

Throughout this book, athletes and climbers share what the practice of yoga has done for their physical health and how it has honed their mental focus. But you don't have to be a professional athlete to benefit. Many climbers are interested in or already practice yoga. Get ready to see how it will give you a context to understand your body while climbing, deepen your appreciation for why you climb, and offer new tools to support your mental and physical health.

HOW TO USE THIS BOOK

This book is intended to be a general guide to the practice of yoga, providing a new perspective and deeper understanding of your body—and how you are impacted when climbing. There are directions for nearly 70 poses with mix-and-match opportunities in 3 complete sequences. As you work your way through this book, you will start to recognize some of the foundational poses. In chapter 3, you will learn about poses that can support the specific stresses your body experiences during a climb, organized by body part and presented as stand-alone poses. In chapter 4, you will discover the benefits of adding a yoga practice to your routine, from developing strength to recovering post-climb, with sequences for each. And in chapter 5, you can apply what you have learned as a setup just before and right after a climb.

In chapters 4 and 5, the poses are presented in sequences (building strength, post-climb recovery, before a climb warm-up, after a climb cool down) that flow from one pose to the next. These sections also provide more detailed information about how to deepen or modify the pose, as well as common challenges and where to focus your attention.

All of these practices are designed for daily use and also for recovery post-climb. In this book you will also learn ways of supporting yourself during the week, including starting a meditation practice, bringing mindfulness to what you eat, managing injury, and approaching your health from a holistic perspective. You'll read through personal stories and hear about research, giving you a deeper understanding of the cultural challenges we all face in taking care of our bodies.

The practice of yoga in the Western world encompasses many styles and philosophical approaches. Climbers looking to expand their yoga practice beyond what I share in this book will get tips on finding a local yoga class and style suited to you—as well as a yoga community—to continue to bring the benefits of yoga into not only their climbing life, but their whole life.

With your purchase of this book, you also get access to our easy-to-use, downloadable cheat sheets for each of the three sequences featured in chapter 4! • Go to our website: www.mountaineersbooks.org/YogaClimb • Download the PDF. • When you open the document on your computer, enter the code "Str3tch13!" when prompted. It's our way of thanking you for supporting Mountaineers Books and our mission of outdoor recreation and conservation.

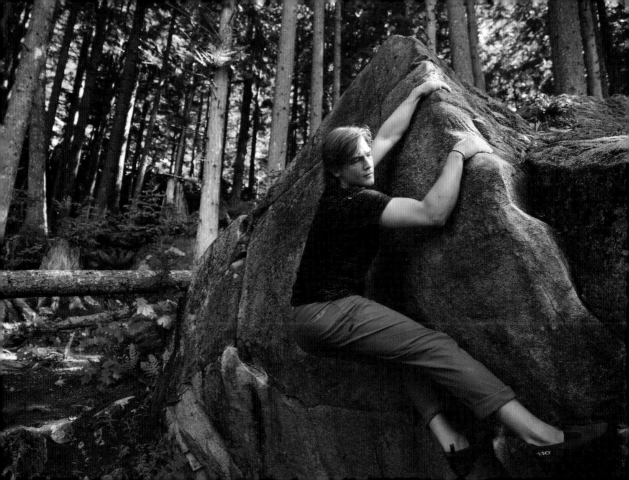

CHAPTER 1
AN INTRODUCTION TO YOGA

YOU HAVE PRACTICED YOGA, even if you didn't know it. You experience yoga when silenced by a sunset—layers of gold, tangerine, and pink streaking across the sky. You feel it when a breeze brushes across your skin while you are climbing a route, as you become aware of both the bigness of the rock wall and focused on the detail of the holds that are the answer to your next move. You light up with yoga when held by someone you love deeply, be it a child, friend, or lover—so close and connected you do not need words.

The word *yoga* means "union," a yoking of body and mind; it is a state of being, a state of unity. Yoga is an ancient, internal practice most widely known for the physical practice of yoga poses, or asana (AH-sah-na). The goal of yoga is to achieve consciousness, or awakening, and the way to do so is in the present moment. How do you get there? Through your physical body, you discover yourself. In yourself, you learn all the answers you have ever needed.

It starts simply, with the connection to the sole of your foot on the floor, to your breath, to your spine. In those moments of awareness of your body, your mind arrives in the present. You may find after practicing, you notice how tight your hips are or become aware of an ache in your lower back. The more you practice, the easier it will be to determine what feels good physically, and what doesn't. You'll learn to differentiate between pain and intensity. You'll understand if you tend to give up when you could instead push yourself—or discover you're the type to push yourself into injury.

YOGA EQUIPMENT

With a few basic tools, you can practice anywhere—at home or on the road. Props are essential to supporting your practice; even experienced yogis rely on them.

» **Mat:** Yoga mats are widely available, ranging from affordable to higher end; the latter tend to offer more padding and grip and are likely to last for years. Mats vary in weight. Most higher-end manufacturers produce lighter mats for travel.
» **Yoga block:** A basic foam or cork block supports your alignment in poses. It also is helpful for seated postures. Note that a block can be used at three different heights.
» **Strap:** A six- or eight-foot strap is useful for multiple poses. For tight shoulders, you can use a strap to bind your hands. A strap can be used to support full relaxation or to intensify some poses.
» **Blanket:** A cozy covering is helpful for a meditation setup and for keeping you warm during savasana, or final rest.
» **Bolster:** A soft bolster is a nice alternative to a block during seated postures.
» **Comfortable, stretchy clothes:** Wear comfortable, stretchy clothes to keep from feeling restricted during your practice.

Through poses, your awareness expands: You notice when you struggle to keep your gaze focused (*drishti*). You see when your mind cries out for you to get out of an intense pose like Frog, a deep hip opener. You find you can last far longer in Warrior 2 than you originally thought—and you realize that you think a lot in this quiet standing power pose!

JUST LIKE EVERY ROUTE or problem is different, dependent on the weather, your climbing buddy, how you feel that day, and your mental state, a yoga practice is the same—a path of exploration, with as many soaring summits and curious valleys as any climb you may encounter. Be playful as you practice, just as you are when you climb. Laugh along the way if you fall over in a balance pose. Instead of being frustrated if you can't get a pose, shrug and smile. There is always another day and another pose. Or slow down to appreciate your own strength, just like how you pause on the wall to puzzle out your next move. See your body for what it is—a powerful vessel to carry you in life and the best teacher you'll ever know.

A BRIEF HISTORY OF YOGA

The spiritual and life-instructive elements of yoga can be found in ancient Indian teachings dating back 5000 years. Patañjali formalized these teachings into the *Yoga-Sutras* about 2000 years ago, creating the seminal text that remains the foundation for yoga. Author Chip Hartranft writes in *The Yoga-Sūtra of Patañjali*, the work "stands as a testament to heroic self-awareness, defining yoga for all time."

Modern yoga bears little resemblance to yoga during Patañjali's time, when postures were focused on seated ones, rather than the athletic poses practiced in gyms and yoga studios today. Yet the study of the Eight Limbs as written in the *Yoga-Sūtras* is the root for today's modern yoga

CREATING A SPACE FOR YOGA AT HOME

....

Create a calm, peaceful environment for yourself at home.
» Use a quiet space that is empty of distractions—no television.
» Shut the door, if you can.
» Let others know not to interrupt you for a set period of time.
» Turn off your cell phone.
» Commit to a set period of time to practice, no matter how short, and stick to it.
» If you prefer to practice with music, keep it in the background.

practice, even as the physical practice and presentation has evolved with Western culture. The teachings of yoga, or union, are still alive because the ancient teachings apply to—and are perhaps needed even more urgently—in modern life.

THE EIGHT LIMBS

The Eight Limbs outlined in the *Yoga-Sūtras* include a practice with eight components. The limbs most familiar to modern day yogis are **asana**, or postures, and **breath work**. Combined, these two limbs form a powerful foundation.

Most people are drawn initially to the physical part of the practice, the asana, for various reasons from health to strength to flexibility. The physical practice is initially the easier part to understand and is a potent component of yoga that gives access to experience the entirety of the practice. Yet the physical practice is only one part of the whole.

BUT THERE ARE MANY elegant ways to approach other elements of the Eight Limbs, as shared by Hartranft. You practice some of them on the wall. Climbers intuitively understand **concentration, or dharana**. By staying present to the challenge of your body and the next move on the rock, you know you can persevere to make the next challenging leap and to climb a route that has eluded you.

The first four limbs emphasize behavior, the physical body, and the development of energetic

THE EIGHT LIMBS

ADAPTED FROM HARTRANFT'S *YOGA-SŪTRAS OF PATAÑJALI*

1. Yamas (five external disciplines, or ethical standards)
   » ahimsa (nonharming)
   » satya (truthfulness)
   » asteya (nonstealing)
   » bramacharya (right use of energy, including sexual)
   » aparigraha (being nonacquisitive)
2. Niyamas (five internal disciplines)
   » saucha (purity)
   » santosha (contentment)
   » tapas (intense discipline or zeal)
   » svadhyaya (self-study)
   » isvara pranidhana (devotion or surrender to pure awareness, or god)
3. Asana (sitting postures)
4. Pranayama (breath regulation)
5. Pratyahara (withdrawal of the senses)
6. Dharana (concentration)
7. Dhyana (meditation or absorption)
8. Samadhi (bliss, self-realization)

awareness. The five **external disciplines**, or the *yamas*, include nonharming, truthfulness, non-stealing, right use of energy (including sexual), and being non-acquisitive. You can practice being truthful at any time, by being honest with yourself and your body on a climb, knowing when you can take on a particularly tough boulder, for example, or listening to your body to know when you need to rein it in. Another limb encompasses the five **internal disciplines**, or the *niyamas*—purity, contentment, intense discipline, self-study, and devotion to pure awareness, or god. You may have experienced contentment when taking off your climbing shoes, stretching out your toes at the end of a long multipitch day, and kicking back with a giant meal at a local diner.

The latter four limbs address the mind and a higher state of consciousness. You may have accessed the practice to **withdraw the senses**, your mind focused on one move at a time, without attachment to the climb, your performance, or the wall. You observe movement and the climb "without desire or judgment," as B. K. S. Iyengar explains in his book, *Light on Life*.

"How can you move toward something that, like Divinity, is already by definition everywhere? A better image might be that if we tidy and clean our houses enough, we might one day notice that Divinity has been sitting in them all along."

—B. K. S. Iyengar, *Light on Life*

There is a limb focused on a meditative experience, or **absorption**, that you may have felt when you climb. When you are on the wall, transfixed by what it will take for you to turn one hip, lift your foot, and stretch your fingertips to the next micro hold above, there is nothing but the wall—you are relaxed, aware, and hypertuned to your body and the experience, like its own meditation. Then there is the limb **samadhi**, the practice of experiencing no distance between you and what is around you, whether it's people or nature, that everyone and everything is the Divine. It's one reason so many of us love being out in nature.

As you focus on yoga poses and breath work, observing your body in new ways, also notice how the practice relates back to all of the Eight

Limbs. The practices are a roadmap for the way you approach any aspect of life—the next climb, an upcoming project at work, or even whether you express appreciation for the people you love. Through the exploration of your physical body and your mind, compassion, gentleness, or joy may arise. Observe the shifts, and see what else is possible.

YOGA FUNDAMENTALS

Yoga starts with awareness. The first layer is the physical one. Through awareness of how your body does basic functions like breath or balance upright during yoga poses, you begin to practice the Eight Limbs.

BREATH

Sometimes, on a hard route, on a hard day, when the next move on the wall feels impossible, you realize you aren't breathing. As you cling by your fingertips to the rock, your breath is the faintest whisper in the background. You realize how tense your face is, how furrowed your brow as you stare at the next hold. You pause, take a full breath in, and exhale it all the way out, trust your feet, and make your move.

Breath is an automatic body function: respiration happens all day long, whether you are awake or asleep. Breath also is a natural filtration system. When you inhale, you draw in fresh air and oxygen; when you exhale, you release carbon dioxide and other toxins.

You don't *need* to pay attention to it. But what happens when you do? Even right now, you may have started to notice your breath. When you do intentional breath work, you connect your conscious mind to a primitive function. In doing so, you activate your parasympathetic nervous system, slowing your heart rate, among other internal functions. After a particularly hard stretch on the wall, breath can make all the difference to take down your heart rate and clear your mind.

Try it for a moment. Take a deep full breath in, pause, then exhale all the air out. Do it three times. You may notice stress or anxiety dissipating. Your heart rate slows; your body relaxes.

Practice breathing off the wall and you'll be more likely to breathe at the moments you need it most. Climber Jay Wyatt says he doesn't always remember to breathe. The constant reminders during yoga teach him to bring it into his sport. "When you're tense on the wall, a couple deep breaths go a long way," he says.

Breath (pranayama) is a fundamental element in yoga. The main breath practice is an ancient one known as *ujjayi* (oo-JAI), or victorious breath. As well-known anatomy expert Leslie Kaminoff writes in *Yoga Anatomy*, "If you take care of the exhalation, the inhalation takes care of itself."

ELEMENTS OF UJJAYI

Enter any room where people are practicing yoga and you will hear ujjayi breath. It's a low, lovely background sound to a practice. The technique requires you to breathe through your nose while constricting your throat. It creates a sound akin to the lapping of ocean waves at the beach. The sound keeps you focused on breathing. Ujjayi also physically directs your breath into the ribs in your back, stretching the intercostal muscles that connect your ribs. Engaging your core lock—addressed later in this chapter—also supports your ujjayi breath.

Breathing is an inherently energetic practice (and there are other styles of breath work beyond ujjayi). You can direct it even more by breathing in an intention that supports you, such as joy or calm, and exhaling something you are ready to shed, like stress or anxiety.

Ujjayi contracts the muscles in your throat and helps you control the speed and depth of your breath—and generates heat. Controlling your breath helps you breathe deeper and more fully. When you first learn ujjayi, you may find either your exhalation or your inhalation is longer than the other. During the practice below, focus on gently balancing them.

Breath Practice

» Find a comfortable seated position, either in a chair or on the floor atop a cushion.
» Sit up straight, and pull your belly button in toward your mid-spine.
» Lift your shoulders to your ears, then relax them down.
» Place your hands around your ribs (fingers in front), circling the front and back of your body.

- » Take a deep breath in through your nose until you feel your ribs expand, open your mouth and exhale with an extended "haaaaa" sound. Keep your belly engaged as you exhale.
- » Take another deep breath in through your nose. This time, keeping your mouth closed for the exhale, repeat the "haaaaa" sound (it will come from your throat) and keep your core engaged. This is ujjayi breath.
- » Repeat. Don't force your breath; let the sound be a whisper, while still breathing deeply.
- » If you need to, gently smooth out your breath until you are breathing evenly in and out. Count to five for each round of inhale and exhale. Do this for one minute.
- » Sit quietly, and observe any shifts in what you feel in your body or your state of mind.

YOUR UJJAYI BREATH IN PRACTICE

When you exert yourself and find it difficult to stay upright in a pose—let alone breathe—you may revert to old breathing patterns and pant through your mouth. Close your mouth! And try again. If you notice you are unable to recover your ujjayi breath, relax into Child's Pose: close your mouth and breathe through your nose until you recover enough to come back to your practice.

"Pranayama is thus the science of breath. It is the hub round which the wheel of life revolves."

—B.K.S. Iyengar, *Light on Yoga*

FOUNDATION

Your feet carry you many thousands of steps a day, and on the wall, they are essential to completing your route. Akin to a climb, in yoga, there is so much more to be discovered in your feet, which connect you to the ground you are walking on, and your hands, which guide you up a wall. Focusing on your feet and hands in your yoga practice will not only stretch and strengthen feet frequently squished by climbing shoes and hands used to gripping rock, it will open up a new appreciation for the connection points between you and the earth.

A yoga practice builds from the ground up. Since many poses start from standing, that means your feet. Yogis practice barefoot to keep the connection of feet to the floor. Notice how sensitive your feet are to sensation by paying attention to the texture of your mat or the floor under the soles of your feet. By practicing barefoot and challenging balance in poses, you will strengthen the muscles deep in your feet and gain more balance and stability.

Wiggle your toes on the floor or inside your shoes. Notice how it brings your attention to your feet. When you do the same with your feet in a yoga practice, standing tall in Mountain Pose, your entire posture changes. You activate new muscles in your legs, and become strong and connected in your lower body. Keep applying the same intention and focus to every part of your body, and you'll soon build up a strong and centered Mountain Pose, the foundational pose of all yoga poses.

In a yoga practice, you spend a significant amount of time on your hands. In Downward-Facing Dog, for example, when you flatten your palms and press the knuckles at the base of your pointer and middle fingers to the floor, your arms straighten and take the stress of the pose out of your elbow joints. It's a small move with a big impact.

Bring one of your hands in front of you. Stretch out your fingers. Notice the space between your fingers. Look at your palm. Look at the back of your hand. Put this book down for a moment and bring your palms together. Press your knuckles at the base of your fingers together and tune in to the sensitivity of your fingertips. Observe the warmth of your skin. Are your palms rough or callused from climbing? Your body senses all of these things without needing your thoughts.

Your hands may be strong from the tight grip needed on the wall. Yoga will teach you to stretch your hands fully. The practice will help you get more mobile in your hands and wrists, as well as your feet, giving you more freedom to move comfortably on and off the wall. Pay attention to your hands and feet throughout the practice, connect them to the ground, and restore their natural energy and strength.

Foundation Feet Practice

Set a timer for one minute, and walk barefoot. Walk mindfully, noticing every part of your foot that comes into contact with the floor. Pay attention to which part of your foot strikes the floor first. Does the entire sole of your foot touch the floor with each step? Observe your toes and how they keep you from falling forward. Notice how your feet hold you up, how sensitive they are to every step. Feel the texture of the floor under your feet. Do your feet tend to rotate in or out? Does your stride change when you pay close attention?

» After one minute, stop and stand with your feet hip-width apart and flat on the floor. Bend from your hips, knees soft, and bring your hands to your feet.
» Bring your thumbs on top of the knuckle at the base of your big toe and press. Keep your thumbs on your big toe knuckle and press your little toe knuckle with your fingers until both knuckles feel evenly connected to the floor.
» Lift the arch of your foot up toward your shins without lifting your big toe knuckle off the ground. Press down into the solidness of your heels.
» Lift your toes up and stretch them out as wide as possible; notice what it feels like to stretch your toes and toe knuckles.

» Keeping space between your toes, settle them back down on the floor. Stand for a moment. Note the texture of the floor, and how the soles of your feet feel.
» Set a timer again. Walk again for one minute with active feet. Observe shifts in your body as you walk.

Foundation Hand Practice

» Come to the floor on your hands and your knees.
» Point your index fingers toward the front edge of your mat. Spread out your hands wide so there is a gap between every finger.
» Lift your fingertips off the floor. Ground the knuckles in your palms flat to the floor; focus on the knuckles under your first and middle finger. Soften your fingers down to the floor. Lift the heels of your hands off the floor so they are vertical to the floor; keep your fingers on the floor. Repeat ten times.
» Turn your hands so your fingers point in toward your knees, thumbs out and palms down toward the floor. Stretch your fingers as wide as they will go. Press the knuckles at the base of your

fingers into the floor as deeply as possible. Lift the heels of your hands off the floor. Press them back down to the floor; it's OK if the heels of your hands don't come all the way down. Repeat ten times.

» Keep your hands turned in toward your knees. Flip to the top sides of your hands, palms facing up with thumbs facing inside of your hands. Keep your fingers on the floor and lift the palms vertically, fingers still on the floor. Press them back down. Repeat ten times.

» Keep your hands in the same position. Curl your fingers in toward your palms as deeply as you can. Release your fingers back to the floor. Repeat ten times.

CORE

Your core is your silent buddy on a climb. When you work from your center, the rest of your body follows, your upper limbs radiating strength from your trunk. You move smoothly and with more control from hold to hold. Your torso contains the key to your climbs, and building endurance will help with stability, mobility, and injury prevention overall.

Luckily, a yoga practice addresses your core strength basically throughout the entire practice. In yoga, *uddhiyana bandha*, or "upward-lifting lock," is used in all poses in the practice. Using your core lock (pulling your belly in toward your spine and up toward your shoulder blades—see the core and root lock sidebar below) supports your lower back, elevates your spine, and engages your back muscles. When using uddhiyana bandha throughout a yoga practice, you are conditioning your belly muscles. Get your core used to engaging, and it will be quicker to engage on the wall.

UDDHIYANA BANDHA ALSO SUPPORTS a deep breath practice. If you are having trouble with your ujjayi breath, engage your core and focus again, extending your inhales and your exhales and breathing into your back ribs.

As the central connecting point in your body, your trunk transfers force from your lower to upper body. Your core works from all sides to protect your spine. If you are struggling with injuries, your trunk is a vital area to take a look. Specific poses will strengthen your trunk. Your oblique muscles

CORE AND ROOT LOCK

To engage your Core Lock, pull your belly button in like you are buttoning a tight pair of pants. Now, lift your belly upward toward your back ribs until your chest lifts. Keep breathing and shift your focus to your front ribs. If the muscles where your front ribs meet are not engaged, your front ribs will pop out. Imagine a little kid sticking their belly forward—cute, but not what you want. When you flare your ribs, you also drop into your middle and lower back.

Wrap your hands around your front rib cage. Pull your fingertips toward each other until the front tips of your ribs squeeze toward each other. Keep your core engaged, and lift your chest up toward the ceiling again. Notice your posture and energy when your belly muscles are fully engaged.

Another less visible action when engaging your core is a lock known as *mula bandha*, your root lock. It is your pelvic floor, and it supports the lift of your core. Essentially, you lift your anus in toward your body similar to the action you take to keep from wetting your pants. Try to lift it without squeezing your inner thighs or butt cheeks.

Mula bandha lifts from the base of your pelvis, pulling in toward the centerline. Since it works from the bottom of your pelvis, the fulcrum for the body, it creates stability energetically and physically, with a calming effect on your nervous system.

along the sides of your abdomen grow stronger in Plank; your lower back and spine builds in belly backbends and your mid-back muscles develop during twists. If you suffer from a sore lower back, a yoga practice will strengthen key muscles in your trunk to help alleviate pain. And no matter how strong your core gets, you will always feel it in poses like Boat!

Core Strength Practice

» Position yourself on your hands and knees to set yourself up for a push-up. Stack your hands right under your shoulders with your fingers spread and your index finger pointed toward the front of your mat.

» Keep your hips just below the height of your shoulders. Pull your belly button in toward your spine, and tip your tailbone toward your feet. Press your hands into the floor. Tuck your toes under, and press your heels firmly away from your body.

» Squeeze your thigh muscles and glutes. Stretch your chest forward akin to sitting up straight. Roll your shoulder blades toward your spine. Lift your gaze toward the front of your mat so that your head is even with your spine. To modify, keep your knees on the floor and lower your hips so your body is level from shoulders to knees.

» Set a timer. Build up to hold for sixty seconds.

CENTERLINE

Your body has a plumb line that keeps you centered when you walk. It uses this centerline to navigate its balance. When you wear a heavy pack or carry a crash pad, your body adjusts to balance itself with this additional weight making your centerline shift—sometimes for the worse when you hopscotch across a stream on your way to a boulder.

During your yoga practice, your body recalibrates balance and strength according to the shape of each pose. Awareness of and understanding of your centerline will give you more access to stability and the natural alignment of each pose. Most of the cues for the poses move your body toward your centerline and your spine to hug your bones in toward your midline. Your spine is where stability lives in your body. The more you access the centerline, the more ease you'll experience in your practice and while climbing.

EQUIPMENT: TWO BLOCKS

» Come to your hands and knees on a mat. Turn a block to the narrowest width and put it between your inner thighs up as high as you can toward your pelvis and squeeze. Place the other block on the floor in front of you, wide and flat. Bring your thumbs to the bottom edge of the block, and the corners of the block into the crease between your thumb and index finger. Your index fingers will point straight ahead.

» Come to Plank, keeping your hands in place at the block. Stack your shoulders over your hands. Lift your legs off the floor. Lower your hips just under your shoulders. Ground your palms into the mat. Lift your head so it's even with your shoulders. Set your gaze in front of your block on the floor.

EXPERIENCE CENTERLINE

» Sag your hips and soften your legs, almost to the point of dropping the block. Notice what happens when you lose your centerline.

» Lift your hips again just below your shoulders. Squeeze your block between your inner thighs firmly. Hug your hands and upper arm bones in toward the block on the floor. Notice the shift in energy through your core and your legs when you hug in toward the center. Do your limbs feel lighter, more aligned, and in sync with your body?

GAZE

For three years, I've taught yoga to kids at the White House Easter Egg Roll. Every year, it feels like more kids say they do yoga at school, or know breathing techniques they learned from their teachers. One year, another yoga teacher filmed a conversation with a kid named Elijah, who said his teachers taught him to practice looking at one spot for one minute at a time. She asked him why he does that. "It helps you concentrate on stuff," he replied. "Like when you're with your friends and you're trying to do your homework. You have to concentrate on your homework."

Well said, Elijah. The same applies to a climb. Have you ever been on a climb where you noticed your mind wandered? It's possible you fell, or got tense, or spent extra energy on a move you could have executed easily otherwise.

Focus and concentration require practice. Yoga poses rely on *drishti* (a simple, focused gaze) to keep your concentration in a pose. Gaze is a foundational part of a yoga practice, and a powerful way to bring concentration into your day. Setting your gaze over and over is a reminder to stay in the present.

You will see cues for your drishti throughout the poses found in this book. By adding drishti and concentration into your life, you may become more productive, plus your mindfulness and your ability to stay present while in conversation may grow exponentially. When combined with breath, drishti also offers release from stress and anxiety.

Drishti Candle Practice

» Light a candle. Set a timer for one minute. Set your gaze on the flame and stay with it. Notice the movement of the flame, what impacts it, how it flickers, flares, and settles. Soften your eyes. Stay focused. Notice if you are tempted to move, and keep your drishti in one spot.

VINYASA FLOW

Vinyasa is the combination of breath and poses, moving in a flow and rhythm with the body. When you connect poses to an inhale or an exhale, you can notice how the inhale supports lengthening and the exhale connects you to the empty space in your lungs and body. Like your drishti, staying focused on your breath requires a certain amount of rigor and discipline. When you get the flow, it's akin to the days you feel ease and grace while climbing. Your feet move smoothly, you waste no energy fumbling for the next move, there is no drama, only transitions from hold to hold with focused power and attention.

I love simple Sun Salutations A and B to open my practice. When I first connect to my breath and my body, I often feel tired, and I move slowly. But as my body warms up, my focus sharpens. I tune into my core, my hands on my mat, and the sound of my breath—much like on a climb, when you start to flex the muscles in your hands and forearms, and your hands remember the sensation of pulling on rock. You might feel stiff and wonder if you were too ambitious about the day ahead. But as you test out the first few moves to

OLIVIA HSU
Boulder, Colorado

Olivia Hsu has been doing yoga almost as long as she has been climbing. Like many climbers, she started to practice because of an injury.

Hsu practices Ashtanga, an intense form of vinyasa flow that requires extraordinary strength and flexibility in the body. Climbing and yoga are similar in that you need both strength and flexibility, she says. If you are flexible enough for a high step but not strong enough to do anything with it, your flexibility doesn't mean anything. The same applies to challenging yoga poses.

Hsu, a professional climber who has been featured on the cover of national magazine *Yoga Journal*, practices five or six days a week. Her two-hour yoga practice is built into her day, like brushing her teeth.

Yoga is so deeply ingrained in her body, she naturally applies it to climbing. Yoga and climbing have a similar rhythm, Hsu says, a cadence that moves between intensity and relaxation. When she is on a difficult stretch of a climb and at her maximum heart rate, she breathes to slow her heart rate down—a technique she applies during difficult yoga poses. "It's like trying but not trying at the same time," Hsu says. "What a paradox."

Many climbers look at yoga as a technique for recovery, but Hsu considers it an excellent training tool. She can drop out of climbing intensely for a month and focus on yoga, and return in relatively good shape, she said. It would not work if she did the opposite, choosing climbing and foregoing her yoga practice.

Yoga has taught her to listen to her body and not be attached to how it feels on any particular day. Some days, she wakes up feeling good and she feels stiff throughout her practice. Other days, she feels sore and her practice is strong. The same applies to climbing. "I've sent projects really tired," she says. "It's like that idea of not being attached to something, not having that expectation."

Hsu started doing yoga for the physical aspect, but over time, the philosophy has settled into her body by application—practicing over and over again. "You just have to do it," she says. "When we practice, our bodies are like a metaphor of our mind."

warm up, your body remembers what it is like to climb. You examine holds, you reach for them, and your confidence grows. Your body is ready for what is ahead.

A flow practice builds heat. Moving through poses in a vinyasa builds strength and also reminds your muscles how to do the poses. The flow requires you to notice when you are lagging with your breath or adding in superfluous movements that take away from the essential combination of pose, inhale, and pose, exhale.

For new practitioners, the art of linking movement and breath can feel elusive. Not all yoga styles include flow, and if you are new to it, vinyasa can feel messy. It may lead to uncertainty about whether you are doing the alignment properly when holding each pose for "one breath," or if you are flowing in sync. It takes time to develop the breath work and the physical strength to move through the poses with alignment and coordination. Be playful with it, notice when you get perfectionist. Stay in the intention of moving with your breath. It will come eventually.

Once you get accustomed to a flow practice and to tapping into your body's strength, a quiet rhythm and peace will come with vinyasa. Your breath begins to enhance each pose as you become experienced. Inhales create space in your physical body, allow you to deepen into your core, and focus on alignment. They are timed for poses that lengthen the spine or expand your energy out like Halfway Lift or stretching your fingers to the ceiling in Warrior.

An exhale creates space by pushing the air out of your lungs for a Forward Fold or to sustain your focus on your Core Lock (see sidebar above). Exhales also allow you to soften and deepen into a pose, supporting your body to stay in a challenging pose longer. Stay in the practice of breath by keeping your focus on how your body moves with your breath.

Basic Vinyasa Practices

» **Seated Vinyasa**: Take a comfortable seat. Rest your hands in your lap. Inhale and circle your arms out wide and up to the ceiling until your palms touch. Exhale and draw your palms down through your centerline to your chest. Repeat this cycle for ten breaths.

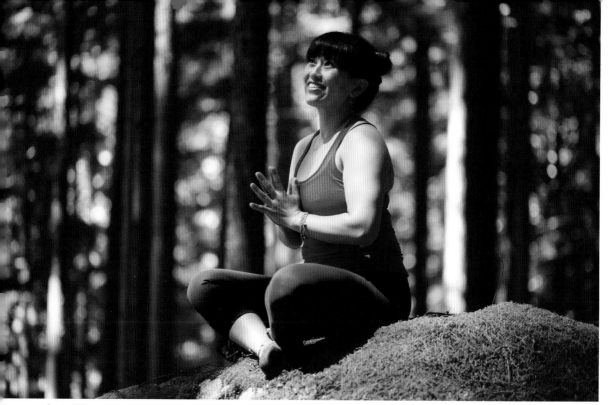

Seated Vinyasa

» **Cat–Cow**: Come to all fours on your hands and knees. Stack your hands underneath your shoulders, with your index fingers pointing to the front of the mat and palms pressed flat into the floor (see photos and instructions on pp. 190–192). Stack your knees underneath your hips. Pull your belly button in, engaging your core. On your inhale, slowly lift your chest forward and up. Tilt your tailbone up toward the ceiling and squeeze your shoulder blades toward each other, keeping your core engaged as your belly dips like a cow. On your exhale, round your spine and your shoulders, pulling your belly up toward the sky and lowering your head and gaze at the floor, like a cat. Move back to Cow on an inhale, and repeat Cat on the exhale. Do this sequence for ten breaths.

MOUNTAIN POSE

Growing up in the Midwest, I remember the first time I saw the stark peaks of the Rockies. I was in high school, and my parents took me to Colorado. I couldn't believe the sheer size and height of the snowy peaks. I craned my neck out the car window, and experienced a scale I didn't know existed until that moment.

Similar to the experience of realizing there is something so much bigger than yourself is Mountain Pose—it connects you to the scale and inspiration of your own physical form. Through the pose, you feel the foundation of your own feet, your strength, your spine, your energy.

All poses wire your body up for healthy, neutral alignment, which supports you as you access your body's full potential. It makes you healthier for long climbs, alerts you to when your body isn't feeling right, and also gives you a better understanding of how to recreate a feeling of alignment and freedom. Like a long, multipitch climb that pushes you to your limit, in Mountain Pose, you can tap into the experience that you are stronger than you can possibly know. You realize how amazing the human body is, and in particular, how strong and powerful you are.

Mountain Pose starts in your feet, stretched broadly on the floor. Once your feet are aligned in a neutral position, your legs connect in, strong and grounded. From there, observe the tilt of your

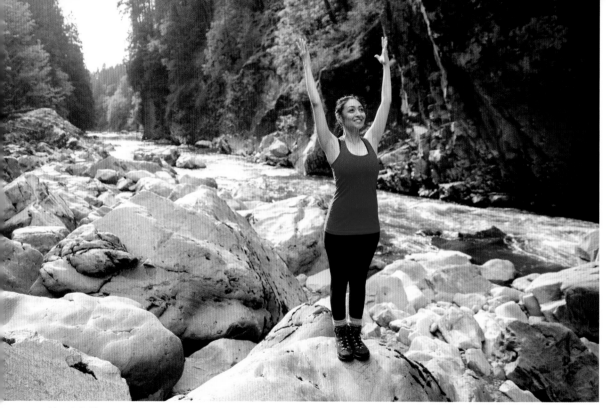

Mountain Pose

pelvis. You now have a foundation to move it into neutral, with the front and back of your pelvis even. Your belly now has more space to squeeze in and lengthen your spine. Pull your shoulder blades toward your spine to lift your chest even higher. Your head can now reach up the same way a mountain peak juts into the clouds. Your breath has more room to expand into your lungs. Practice the pose to experience the shift in energy and perspective possible from such a simple, essential place.

Mountain Pose Practice

Each of the cues in this pose builds upon another; layer them in one by one.

» Stand on a mat with your bare feet directly under your hips, your arms loose by your sides.
» Point your toes straight ahead, and bring the outer edges of your feet parallel with the edges of your mat; you may observe a slight pigeon-toe. Lift your toes and connect with the four corners of your feet to the mat. Soften your toes back to the floor.

» Lift the arches of your feet, and with all four corners of your feet evenly grounded, press your outer shins out until you feel your legs engage, then spiral your inner ankles toward the back of your mat. Energetically, drive your outer ankles down to the floor.
» Squeeze your thigh muscles to the bone. If your knees became stiff, soften the joints slightly.
» Tilt your tailbone down toward the floor. Gently pull in your belly button to engage your core. Squeeze your front ribs toward each other.
» Roll your shoulders up to your ears, then soften them down away from your ears. Pull your upper arm bones toward your shoulder blades to engage your shoulders.
» Send breath into your ribs in your mid-back.
» Let your hands relax by your sides, and spin your palms to face forward.
» Lift the crown of your head up toward the sky to lengthen your neck. Soften your jaw.
» Set your gaze on one point.
» Take ten deep ujjayi breaths.
» Observe what it feels like to ground your feet and notice the rise of energy along your spine

and center. Experience how it radiates from your center out through your fingers and up through the crown of your head. Note what it is like to connect to your physical body and the present moment through Mountain Pose.

INTEGRATE: WORK FROM THE BONES

In climbing, you learned early on to rely on your skeleton. You figured out quickly that hanging with your arms halfway bent tired out your arms. You learned to rely on straight arms and your ligaments and tendons rather than muscles that fatigue quickly.

Integration in yoga works the same way. Mountain Pose teaches you to work from your bones. When you stack your ankles, knees, and hips over the four corners of your feet, your foundation becomes more stable. When you pull your belly in and lower your tailbone toward the earth, your thigh bones pull into your pelvis. Your deep psoas muscle and glutes work together to keep your lower body balanced. Rather than working the superficial muscles, you learn to work in an integrated way into your body's center—ideal for both yoga and for climbing.

You also want to work into the bones in your upper body where it can be easy for climbers to lose integration. When you hug your shoulder blades toward each other, you fire the lower part of your trapezius muscles, which draws the shoulders down and lifts your chest. That same movement has your upper arm bones pulling in to your shoulder blade, which works into the muscles that connect your shoulder blades to your spinal column.

The alignment cues in yoga teach you how to work from your bones and into your center-line, which will deepen your understanding of integration. By challenging your body to access integration in various directions through the poses, your understanding of how to work from your body's skeleton will expand not only in yoga practice but in direct translation to how you tackle the wall, offering new freedom and strength as you climb.

MEDITATION FUNDAMENTALS

Meditation is a practice to train your mind to be present. There are many techniques, and meditation and contemplative practices are found in almost all spiritual traditions, including Christianity, Islam, and Judaism, although it is probably most closely associated with Buddhism.

Like yoga, meditation requires practice. The goal isn't necessarily to relax, but the benefits can be experienced that way. Studies have shown that when you meditate, you lower your blood pressure, blood cortisol levels, and your heart rate. You improve your blood circulation, sweat less, have less anxiety . . . the list goes on.

WHY MEDITATE?

More people than ever are curious about the benefit of a meditation practice. Meditation's growing popularity has led to robust scientific studies focused on the impact it has on the brain and the body. Various recent studies have shown it has cognitive and mental benefits. The magazine *Scientific American* devoted a cover story to the topic called "Mind of the Meditator" in November 2014. In it, the writers noted that brain scans of experienced meditators demonstrated that the practice has a noticeable impact on how their brains are wired. Like a person learning to play an instrument, experienced meditators are able to develop new areas of their brains. They can achieve a focused state of mind with little effort, much like an expert musician or athlete can immerse in a performance with ease.

The studies discuss various types of meditations—such as focused-attention meditation that brings awareness to a physical action like breath; mindfulness or open-awareness meditation that might focus on sight or sound, and not becoming attached to any particular perception or thought; and compassion meditation, when the meditator focuses on feelings of unconditional love and compassion toward others. Meditation has four distinct cycles identified by researchers—time when the mind wanders, a moment when you become aware of the distraction, a period when you reorient your attention, and then the period you resume focused attention.

A study on focused-attention meditators showed they were less likely to react or get distracted when interrupted; they were more able to stay vigilant. Those who focused on open-awareness meditation had improved perception, with depressed patients better managing negative thoughts or feelings and a reduced chance of relapse in some. The compassion meditation helped meditators share the feelings of other people without becoming emotionally overwhelmed, particularly helpful for people in caregiver roles.

Meditation also brings lasting change to brain function, from the levels of stress people experience and an ability to stay calm in the face of stress to an improved immune system and resilient brain cells. Observing an eight-week study of active meditators, Harvard researchers found that brain matter grew in regions of the brain associated with learning, cognition, memory, emotional regulation, empathy, and compassion.

LEARNING TO MEDITATE

A daily meditation practice is a powerful point of connection and is key to understanding some of the deeper qualities of yoga. In Patañjali's time, yoga consisted of mostly seated poses, with a focus on meditation.

Be kind to yourself when starting out, and playful too. Start with five minutes in the morning as soon as you wake up, and sit for five minutes again before you go to bed. Once you are in the routine of bookending your day with meditation, increase the time up to thirty minutes morning and night. Give yourself thirty days to create a meditation practice and see the results.

When you start this practice, your mind will wander. That's OK. Part of the practice is to notice your thoughts. You will not empty your mind, per se. You will initially notice you are thinking, rather than present. Meditation is a practice of return, and even when it does not feel like it is working, trust that it is. Just as your climbing gets stronger with every return to the wall, the more frequently you sit in meditation, the more you will experience greater ease, focus, and less reactivity throughout your day.

"However beautifully we carry out an asana, however flexible our body may be, if we do not achieve the integration of body, breath, and mind, we can hardly claim that what we are doing is yoga. What is yoga after all? It is something that we experience inside, deep within our being."

—T. K. V. Desikachar, *The Heart of Yoga*

CREATING A SPACE
FOR MEDITATION

Creating a comfortable setup for your meditation practice is important for making it a routine. Find a quiet space in your home where you won't be disturbed. Set yourself up with the following props:

» **Meditation cushion:** There are many suppliers of meditation cushions, but you can use any cushion in your house. Use a large cushion for the base to support your ankles, with a smaller cushion set on top that elevates your hips above your knees and makes it easier to sit for longer stretches. You can sit with your legs crossed or with your shins on either side of your smaller cushion.

» **Chair:** If it is challenging for you to sit on a low cushion, sit on a chair. Sit on the front half of the chair away from the back in an upright posture. Prop your feet up if the chair cuts into the back of your legs. Place a cushion or other support behind your back as needed.

» **More props:** During meditation, you may prefer to fold your hands in your lap. One option is to place a cushion or blanket in your lap to keep your hands propped up comfortably. Wrap a blanket around your shoulders for warmth for longer meditations.

» **Altar:** Adding an altar can create a sense of ritual around your meditation practice. Use a small table or get creative. Place treasured items, such as small tokens from loved ones, a candle, or fresh flowers, on the altar.

Lastly, do not underestimate the importance and clarity provided by the daily ritual of meditation. By creating and establishing a ritual to support your own health—and returning to the ritual even if you miss a day—you put your well-being first. Just as you must commit to repeatedly working on a climb that challenges your skill and technique, commit to the practice of meditation. Experience for yourself its impact on you and those around you.

WHEN IS THE BEST TIME TO MEDITATE?

....

Meditation is traditionally practiced in the early morning right when you wake up, and in the evening before you go to bed. Meditating both morning and night bookends your day with a contemplative, quiet space. That said, if you need to squeeze it in, meditating midday is better than skipping out completely!

Breath Meditation Practice

» Sit on a cushion or in a chair. Set a timer for five minutes.
» Close your eyes. Note the feeling of your feet and ankles against the floor. Walk your awareness up your legs to your hips. Stack your vertebrae and sit up straight. Tilt your chin parallel to the floor to lengthen the back of your neck. Bring your awareness to your nose.

» Notice the in and out of your breath over your upper lip. Do not try to control your breath. Pay attention to the natural state of how your body breathes.
» Note how your breath may be cool on the way in and warm on the way out. Focus on the feeling of air passing through your nostrils.
» When you notice your mind wandering, note you have wandered and bring your attention back to your breath. Focus again on your breath coming in and out.

Walking Meditation Practice

If all this talk about sitting sounds uncomfortable, consider a walking meditation practice, most closely associated with the Buddhist tradition. While you will be moving no farther than the distance across your living room, it is a powerful mindfulness practice. (Hint: It's also a practice you can fit in on your way to your next outdoor climb or bouldering session!)
» Find a spot in your home where you can walk ten paces in one direction without any obstacles. Set a timer for ten minutes.

» You can do this practice with or without shoes. Stand still for a moment and close your eyes. Feel the weight of your body over your feet. Notice the bones of your feet.

» Start to walk, focusing lightly on each step. Observe the muscles your body uses to take a step. Pay attention to your feet as you walk. Move slowly, feeling every part of your body as you go.

» When your mind wanders, bring it back to your feet. When you turn around, note what has to happen in your body to turn. Continue your mindful focus on walking.

Mantra Meditation Practice

In a mantra meditation, you focus your mind on a phrase. *So hum* is a basic mantra meditation—it means "I am that" in Sanskrit.

» Sit on a cushion or in a chair. Set a timer for five minutes.

» Close your eyes. For five rounds of breath, notice the natural inhales and exhales of your breath.

» Focusing on your inhale, say the word "so" to yourself. On your exhale, say "hum." Repeat. Observe if your mind wanders to your body or other thoughts, and return to the mantra.

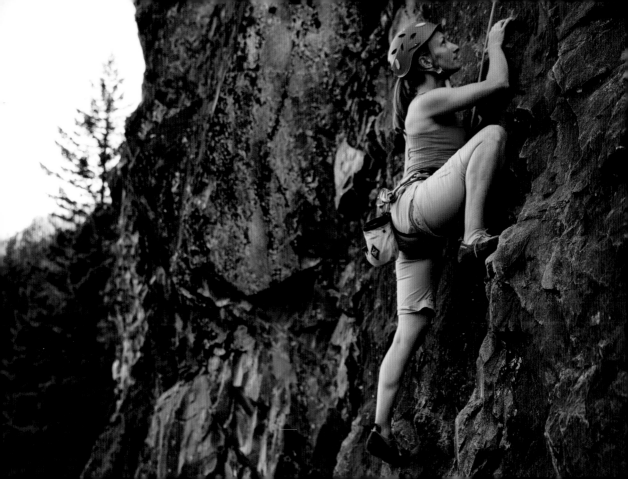

CHAPTER 2
THE BENEFITS OF YOGA

"Yoga says we must deal with the outer or most manifest first, i.e., legs, arms, spine, eyes, tongue, touch, in order to develop the sensitivity to move inward. This is why asana opens the whole spectrum of yoga's possibilities."

—B.K.S. Iyengar, *Light on Life*

AT ITS HEART, YOGA is a multidimensional and transformative practice. It has immense physical benefits, and those are the ones you learn first. Yoga poses help you become strong, flexible, and graceful. Your body awareness expands, while your endurance builds, which comes in handy while contemplating how to arrange your hips and limbs for your next move on the wall.

The physical lessons also are the gateway to the deeper mental ones, which is what ultimately change lives. It's why I practice and teach yoga.

In this chapter, you will learn more about the physical strength, balance, and stability available through a regular yoga practice, in addition to the ways it can support you mentally to sort through whatever challenges life decides to throw your way that day. You'll learn new ways to look at injury and how a yoga practice can help you manage and prevent injury as well as rehabilitate.

THE PHYSICAL BENEFITS
A strong, focused practice can echo a long, arduous day of climbing and the reward of exhausted delight that comes from testing your body's physical

limits. You may start your climb distracted, thinking about how hard the route ahead may be. But after hours of moving your body up and across a rock wall, you have forgotten about your earlier concerns; you can feel your feet, hands, and breath.

In yoga, your attention is similarly focused on the feeling of the mat under you, the experience of inhaling and exhaling, with your drishti focused on one point. You can experience the potent mix of physical work and a sense of calm and connection to something bigger than yourself, much like the experience of being on the wall.

Yoga also brings your attention to your thoughts more readily. You notice you are babbling to yourself, and you rely on your breath, gaze, and physical alignment to turn your focus instead to the present. You've likely figured this out when climbing. Climbing is multidirectional, requiring twists, open hips, and good body awareness. When you are strong and mobile, with a deep understanding of how your body moves in space, you are freed up to take on more technical routes. You know that if you don't stay present with your body and what's happening, that's when you miscalculate, and perhaps fall.

Above all other types of movement, yoga opens me to a deep, physical awareness. When I am nursing an injury, I go to yoga. There, I can breathe, observe rather than push through, and settle the panicked thoughts that launch when something doesn't feel right physically. If I need to take my practice down a notch, I do. Yoga taught me that pushing constantly does not always take me where I need to go, and it's the place I return when I need to get grounded.

Listening to your body is important for anyone, but particularly athletes. Your body endures wear and tear from intense climbs, not to mention arduous approaches with packs loaded with ropes and the gear needed for climbing. Effort is your middle name. Yoga will build more balance into your body with deep layers of stability in your core and long holds that stabilize your joints. A yoga practice also can teach you the importance of lowering the physical intensity and how to add in a restorative yoga practice to serve your body's need to soften and relax rather than muscle through.

Plus, it can be hard to make enough time to climb *every* day. A yoga practice is another way to access the layered benefits experienced on a climb.

The following physical benefits range from the ones you may know, such as flexibility, to ones you haven't considered, like deeper body awareness.

THE HAZARDS OF SITTING

The first time I observed adults squatting was in Beijing, China. It was the mid-1990s, and people squatted everywhere—street corners, Tiananmen Square, the Great Wall of China. Their squat was deep, their heels stayed on the ground. They looked relaxed. My American friends and I tried to emulate them, but after just a few moments, we would grimace and stand up.

Many years of yoga and fitness later, I know the squat is a natural and essential resting position (and movement) for the human body. Observe toddlers. They squat to look at something on the ground, or to communicate with a friend—it doesn't occur to them that it is uncomfortable, because for them, it is not.

Many Americans spend the day with their hips in a static 90-degree position, either in a chair or in a car. Once you hit your school years, where you spend the day at a desk, most of you lost your squat or no longer felt comfortable in it. That also may mean you lose some strength for standing up, and mobility in your hips and lower back. If you struggle to get out of a chair, you most likely end up staying there, a perpetual challenge as people age.

According to a report from the *Washington Post* about the health hazards of sitting, your brain function slows down when you don't have fresh blood moving through it from physical activity. Sitting leads to a strained neck, sore shoulders and back, tight chest, tight hip flexors, and a weak core and glutes. It can lead to a weak spine and bad back, to poor circulation and soft bones from a lack of activity. Extended sitting can lead to high blood pressure, a greater risk of heart disease, and an overproductive pancreas, which can lead to diabetes and a greater risk of colon, breast, and endometrial cancer. Are you convinced yet?

It's important to take breaks from sitting by standing periodically and changing position.

Some people set timers every twenty to thirty minutes at work to remind them to stand up and get blood flowing back into their legs. It's also worth noting that your body is completely capable of reclaiming its squat. Follow the Thirty-Day Squat Challenge below!

THIRTY-DAY SQUAT CHALLENGE

Created by movement leader Ido Portal, this challenge is to bring back your squat. You don't need to do all ten minutes in one stretch, but set out to squat ten minutes a day for thirty days. Set a timer to keep track throughout the day. When it gets too intense, stand up. See how you feel about your body, mobility, and squat ability by the end of the month.

Note: If you have trouble getting into a full squat, you can practice lowering into a chair without sitting all the way onto the seat, hovering until you get strong and open enough to go into a full squat. Or, place a mat or blanket under your heels.

MOBILITY

When I meet someone new and tell him I teach yoga, it often prompts a confession—he doesn't do yoga. Often, he will follow up with a second confession, brow furrowed, that he is terribly inflexible. I counter the confession with my own—I was barely able to touch my toes when I started practicing, but I can now.

You could too (if you can't yet), if you were to practice and access your body's natural ability. The heavens will not open up when you touch your toes, but when your joints move in all the ways available to your body, and your muscles become more pliable, your body is capable of movements including squats, twists, flexing, or extending to touch your toes. Access all of these directions, and you can step higher to the next hold, rotate your hips with ease while climbing, and perhaps even squat easily.

Certain kinds of repetitive movement naturally tighten up your body. Take hiking (which many climbers do if only to get to a favorite wall): It requires your body to move in a similar direction, often for a long time. Your body largely moves in one plane of motion. When you carry a heavy pack loaded with ropes and other gear, or your crash pad, the impact is even more intense. And climbing itself tends to work certain muscles repetitively. If you don't vary the way you move, your hip flexors and hamstrings get tighter. Your lower back and hips take the brunt of your pack weight. Stress and anxiety also accumulate in your physical body, showing up for most people as tightness in their shoulders, and furthering issues with your lower back and hips.

More than that, if you don't challenge your body to do all it is capable of, you limit both your understanding and your range of possibility. The goal with a yoga practice, or any kind of movement, truly should be to experience your body at its optimal, its healthiest, and most energetic.

The key is listening to your body. If you're tight, that means being kind and working slowly into stretches. If you're very open, that means not becoming dependent on your flexibility in poses. You *can* overstretch, especially if you're stretching where the muscle begins, which pulls on tendons and other connective tissue. "Pay attention to stretch into the target muscle itself," says Leslie Kaminoff in *Yoga Anatomy*.

Mobility is key to restoring your body from the intensity of a climb. A yoga practice supports multiple approaches toward mobility. Most people associate flexibility with static stretching.

During Half Pigeon, it takes a full minute before the muscles around the piriformis, a deep hip muscle, relax and the piriformis begins to lengthen, Kaminoff writes. The experience can bounce back and forth between intensity and a deep release.

Yoga poses also include active stretches, known as dynamic stretches, when you contract an opposing muscle to open your muscles safely. For example, engaging your thigh muscles will support flexibility in your hamstrings, opening them more effectively. You also lengthen muscles by contracting in moves like lifting one leg off the floor while in Downward-Facing Dog. In a vinyasa practice, when you repeatedly move through similar poses, muscles stretch over time as they warm up. Your body is doing constant active stretches at the beginning of your practice, contracting some muscles to lengthen other tissue.

Many people experience some form of tightness in their hips and their shoulders. Sitting is a major factor for both. Slumping while sitting also puts pressure on the trapezius, the muscle that connects your neck and shoulders. Your chest curls forward and muscles contract. Also, for people who only ever walk or run, their muscles become accustomed to that same motion and direction.

You may be surprised by how many parts of your body open up through a yoga practice. Your ankles become more flexible with Downward-Facing Dog and squats. Your feet strengthen during balancing poses, translating to greater stability when balancing on your big toe on a hold. You learn to engage your shoulders even more on the wall, tapping into the various muscles in your back rather than relying on your chest, shoulders, and arms to pull yourself up. Yoga poses also include twists to relax tight muscles in your trunk and keep your spine healthy. Backbends open up your chest and heart area, teaching you to release tension that accumulates in your shoulders from climbing.

Your body can release tension through a regular breath practice, which ultimately allows your body to open up. When you work into mobility, you can experience the full freedom of range of motion for climbing and life.

STRENGTH AND STABILITY

The physicality of a yoga practice offers you insight into where your strengths reside, and where you can focus to build needed strength. Holding poses, in particular, requires your body to adapt to what's happening in the moment. Staying in Warrior poses strengthens stabilizer muscles around your hips, knees and ankles, while pausing in Plank stabilizes your wrists, hands, shoulders, and core.

Creating stability in a yoga practice begins at your foundation—your feet. Activate your feet, and your leg muscles will light up, stabilizing your knee and hip joints. Move into your core and shoulders, and you create stability throughout. The more you practice, the more you strengthen different muscles. Your body loves to cheat, and will depend upon the strongest muscle in the body rather than engaging the proper muscle for good alignment. In the standing pose Warrior 2, for example, people often let their front knee cave in and hip jut out, allowing their stronger thigh muscle to compensate for weak glutes or tight hips. By centering your front knee over your ankle and pulling your front thigh bone into your hip socket, you strengthen your outer hip and butt muscles and create more stability around your hip.

All yoga poses call for core engagement throughout the practice and doing so supports your lower back, elevates your spine, and engages your back muscles, all of which you use on a climb.

Yoga also varies the type of movement your body is accustomed to. Rather than the constant emphasis on pulling yourself up the wall in climbing, you focus more on pushing in yoga, which strengthens your bones. With a regular practice, you will notice over time as you get stronger in your core and shoulders, holding Plank—the beginning of a push-up—will not be as hard as it once was, though I can't promise it will ever be easy.

You'll learn to access and stabilize your shoulders so you can access the strong muscles of your back instead of relying on the ligaments in your shoulders. You'll feel your ankles and feet get stronger. You'll experience release and freedom in locked-up hands and wrists. You'll learn to open your chest, relieving years of built-up tightness.

BALANCE

When a practitioner, Marie, first came to me at age seventy-seven, she had trouble standing on one foot. During balancing poses, she would grit her teeth, a look of determination in her eyes. She wanted to do them over and over, occasionally ignoring me when I gently suggested we move on. She taught me a thing or two about discipline—she stopped wearing shoes at home to help her feet get stronger; she practiced Tree while she brushed her teeth; she requested balancing poses every week so she could show me how much she was improving.

After a couple months of weekly yoga sessions combined with her daily regimen, she came in one day and told me that for the first time in years, she was able to pull her pants on, one leg at a time—while standing on one foot. The smallest triumphs can be the biggest breakthroughs, and it was huge for her.

Your body's ability to balance is based on an intricate system including vision, inner balance function in your ears, your core, and legs. Balance is a critical function that runs in the background all day. You don't notice, but your eyes take in the horizon, your ears calculate when your head moves, and your core and feet adjust to movement. Your brain is the coordinator, syncing all of this to keep you upright. It knows how to adjust when you shift your weight from one foot to another to reach for the next hold.

PROPRIOCEPTION

Proprioception is your brain's understanding of where your body is in space. Your body learns balance sensing where your body parts are in relation to each other and gauging strength and movement through muscles, tendons, and your joints.

When you learn a new skill, your body picks up new elements of movement. The more you ask of your body, the more your brain forms circuits between existing neurons to meet the new demands. Proprioception is what allows you to walk in the woods after dusk with a headlamp. It's how you can run without looking at your feet. It's why we feel awkward doing a new, unfamiliar activity—

remember clinging anxiously to holds on the easiest route the first time you tried to climb? Over time, your body has adapted to climbing, understanding intuitively how to shift weight over your feet as you move up a wall.

Challenge your body's sense of space with new activities that are out of your comfort zone. If you don't dance, try a new dance class. If you're not a trained dancer, you might notice how tough it is to coordinate your hands, feet, and torso to the beat. It might feel nearly impossible. But if you keep going back to the class, and practicing the steps over and over, your body starts to learn them. Suddenly, the spin on one foot combined with the stomp of another, is possible. You have just built new circuits for your brain and body.

If you don't challenge your body's ability to balance, you lose it, says Chris Morrow, a physical therapist. The older you get, the less likely you are to test your balance out of fear of falling; one-third of people older than 65 fall every year.

One simple strategy anyone can do to improve balance is to take away one of the essential systems, like sight, Morrow recommends. You can practice your balance in a Tree pose in chapter 3. Another is to focus on the parts of your body that coordinate balance. Notice your feet. See what happens when you scrunch your toes, and your foot arches. Practice lifting all of your toes and setting them back on the floor. Rise up onto the balls of your feet and balance there, then walk. Lift the balls of your feet above your heels, balance, and walk. All of these small movements bring attention to our feet, and you'll notice how the parts work together.

Climbers constantly challenge their body's ability to shift weight from one foot to the next and stay balanced; your body becomes adept at weight transfer. A yoga practice challenges balance in other ways, including playing with sight and inner ear balance by moving your head in different directions. It develops your core, a critical element of balance that will only improve your agility on the wall. But even doing simple standing poses, where you place your feet on the ground at various distances, will deepen your body awareness and challenge your center of gravity.

Many poses strengthen your butt muscles and outer hips, which play a major role in balance. Balancing poses where you stand on one leg shift a key element of your foundation. When your center of gravity moves over one foot instead of two, your body adapts, and you strengthen both your grounded foot and your core. The more you do it on the ground, the simpler it will feel when you are balancing on a tiny foothold.

You might find that your standing foot cramps as it relies on deeper ligaments and tendons that keep your foot stable. With different positions for your upper leg, torso, and arms, your body must figure out new ways to keep you upright.

You also can play with taking away sight in your yoga practice. Start out in a standing Mountain Pose, your eyes closed. Notice how your body sways, adjusting to balance until your pelvis centers itself over your feet. Next, close your eyes in Warrior 2 (see Strength Practice I). Your awareness of your feet grows, and you notice how important it is to engage your core so you don't fall over.

Experiment with eyes closed during Tree pose, and see how much you rely on your eyes to stay upright. Next, observe how your inner ear balance works. Stand in Mountain Pose and turn your head slowly side to side, and notice what happens as your body adjusts. The longer you practice and the more stable your balance gets, the more playful you can be.

STEPH DAVIS
Moab, Utah

Steph Davis started doing yoga out of necessity. Her back had seized up from climbing and trail running, and she had pulled a tight hamstring on a heel hook. When her hamstring healed, she knew she had to change something. "Dammit, I'll have to stretch," she remembers thinking. "It will be terrible."

It was the mid-1990s. She picked up *Light on Yoga*, a foundational text by master teacher B. K. S. Iyengar that outlines the essential elements of the practice and poses.

She did yoga at home, holding poses to see what would happen. She noticed the poses often felt difficult at first, but if she held one long enough, her muscles would release. She could translate that directly to climbing: as her body relaxed in uncomfortable yoga poses, it would do the same in a resting stance on the wall. Her back stopped hurting.

Her muscles are now used to relaxing in the middle of an awkward resting stance. "Like anything, if you train something, it just happens," she said.

One day, she read the introduction to *Light on Yoga*. She realized yoga poses were a pathway and training to meditate. The philosophy resonated with her approach to climbing, and her search for a feeling of flow and expansion. Yoga helped her find her direction, she says.

Davis has been climbing for more than twenty years, and climber culture can feel focused on sending the hardest possible route. But that is not why Davis climbs, despite the fact that she is one of the most famous names in climbing as the first woman to free climb the Salathe Wall on El Capitan in Yosemite National Park and the second woman to free climb El Capitan in under twenty-four hours. "I couldn't really care less what I 'achieve,'" she says. "It's more I want to be experiencing these ideas in a physical way that I have."

Like other climbers, she has given in to thinking she doesn't have enough time to do yoga. Early on, her practice sometimes lasted one minute. Now, she might practice for six minutes, or thirty.

Some days, she is motivated to practice to keep her lower back healthy. Other times, she meditates. "The fact you're going through physical motion, your brain is going to go into more meditative state—really the idea of yoga," she said. "It's not just exercise."

EASE AND RECOVERY

One of the essential yoga teachings is ease. In the *Yoga-Sūtras*, there's a teaching called *sthira sukham asanam* (STEE-rah SOO-kum AH-sa-nam). Basically, it means combining steadiness and ease.

Fun and laughter is a surefire way to invoke ease, especially when students are cursing me under their breath during a long Warrior 2. I often tease my students for being Type A (it takes one to know one), and ask them to observe if they are being overzealous. I can spot those students from across the room—their arms and legs shake, their gaze is like a laser beam drilling a hole into the wall, and they avert their eyes when I suggest they soften their shoulders or jaw to relax into a pose.

But once those students learn to soften, they are often surprised. That is the moment when you can hold a pose longer than you thought. When you take a Chair pose, and you feel your feet, legs, hips, and core resisting gravity, you may still wish for nothing else on this earth but for the pose to end. You also notice that it's possible to deepen your breath, set your gaze, and stay focused. Like the moment when you think you're almost there on a multipitch climb, and then realize you still have another pitch to go—instead of thinking grimly that you'll never make it, you take a deep breath, let go of thinking about how much longer you've got, and you keep going. You practice being present with your body.

The more you relax in a pose and the more your brain can focus on the muscles that hold you there, the better your body understands which muscles to engage and which ones to relax. You don't need to knit your eyebrows in *any* pose, trust me. This softer approach will serve you everywhere, particularly in your approach to climbing. Treat each climb as a moment-by-moment practice. Notice where you can soften and relax as you puzzle through the next move. In the big picture, notice the impact of a relentless drive to reach the next level. It may take you far, but it can come at a great cost as well, in the form of injury or never allowing your body and brain time to come down from an intense adrenaline high.

The next level of ease is supporting your body in release and recovery. If you spend most of your time in intense activity, your nervous system stays in a constant state of stress and tension. Physical therapist Chris Morrow advises that people take on calming exercises for overall health and balance. If your body feels happy, safe, and secure, rather than stressed and anxious, it will perform better.

Adding in a yoga practice dedicated to recovery is important for everyone. In practices designed to help your body relax, and stretch out tight hips and shoulders, you may notice earlier if something is not working properly. Recovery and ease is the path to understanding your body and giving it space to heal and bounce back for the next weekend on the wall.

BODY AWARENESS

Understanding your body starts at the granular level—the sensation of your feet on the floor, the feeling of your ribs expanding and contracting while you breathe. The more you focus on feeling the sensations in your body, the more you will understand how your body moves in space, or proprioception (see sidebar above).

Yoga poses deepen your understanding of where your body is in space and how to maneuver on a microlevel of awareness. Alignment teaches you to feel the difference between pitching your pelvis, shaped like a bowl, forward and a neutral pelvis, where the front and back are even. You might notice you always stand with your pelvis tipped forward, your core slack, contributing to a sore lower back.

The better you know your body and how it moves in space, the deeper your understanding of poses and alignment will be, and the more it will serve you in life anywhere. You'll notice which muscles are strong, and which ones could use some work. You'll trust your body to do what you ask it to do, essential for any climber. You'll feel free to rotate more, using your hips in new ways to keep yourself close to the wall and access different holds. You'll know how to keep your body healthy, safe, and strong.

MIKE PAPCIAK
Berkeley, California

Thirty years into climbing, Mike Papciak takes a slower view of climbing than he once did. In his twenties, when he was a competitive climber, his climbing was impatient. Now, he looks at a route as an opportunity to study the way his body moves. He calls his climbing "yoga bouldering."

Rather than doing a crux move where he falls into connective tissue in his funky shoulder and hopes it doesn't tear, he says, he focuses on moving safely and well. "My climbing has become this beautiful way to relax," he says. "Let me go out and feel good in my body, feel correct in my body, and use climbing as my tool to knit my shoulder together even better."

He was no longer climbing professionally, and he had an office job and a kid. His body was aching and felt stiff, and he wanted that to change. His wife was going to yoga, and he decided to try it out.

Papciak was mesmerized by the Iyengar practice, which focuses on holding poses for long periods, and he liked the attention teachers and practitioners applied to their bodies. He appreciated the absence of music and the slower pace.

Now in his late forties, Papciak still practices yoga for ten minutes a day. His practice consists of four poses that he has learned from private sessions over the years—a twist, a forward fold, a traditional headstand, and Downward Facing Dog, which he calls an excellent education in shoulder rotation. He likes spending time in a pose, investigating how his body feels, and seeing what shifts.

Now a bodyworker doing massage therapy, he calls really good yoga with an experienced teacher "one of the best medicines for the body I have seen." Yoga is excellent cross-training for athletes, he says, and while some of his climbing buddies say they don't have time for yoga, he thinks one day all climbers will consider it indispensable, like fingerboard training.

Papciak says good bodywork is like taking out the garbage, working the rotation of joints and mechanics to wipe your body's chalkboard clean. Pulling as hard as you can with your shoulders at crazy angles is "scribble." Yoga, however, teaches you to move in healthy ways and in good alignment. "If you leave my office with a clear chalkboard, go take a really good yoga class and get some good penmanship on the chalkboard," he says.

A STUDY BY RESEARCHERS at the University of Miami, Florida, discovered that instructors and advanced yoga practitioners engage different muscles than do newcomers to yoga or even practitioners with three years of experience or more. In some poses, for example, instructors used the deltoid muscles in their back in standing forward folds, Downward-Facing Dog, and in Warrior poses. Your deltoids stabilize your shoulders, and those with experience have learned over years of practice to engage while folding to deepen the fold. Newer practitioners struggled to use those muscles. More experienced yogis also were more likely to engage their calf muscles during Halfway Lift and Warrior 1, which stabilizes the ankle, and allows for deeper forward folds and deeper knee bends—an important area of strength for your climbing foundation.

As you practice and focus on alignment, your body will understand how to connect to the bigger, stronger muscles that best support a pose. With deeper body awareness, you also will notice when something feels off and realize it's time to modify until your body heals, rather than pushing through. A consistent yoga practice teaches you the difference between pain and potential injury, and an intense, challenging practice pushes you to the edge of your strength.

MANAGING AND PREVENTING INJURY

An injury can happen before you know it. One of my biggest lessons happened at a rock climbing gym. I lifted my foot for the next hold, and my hip did a little pop. I ignored it—against my own intuition and everything I knew about moving in an integrated, stable way. I stepped onto the next hold and pressed down into my foot with all of my weight. The sudden pain in my groin shocked me. I spent one full week on the couch, barely moving. Even after a couple of weeks, I couldn't practice most yoga poses. It took three weeks before I began to recover.

As you push your body's limits, you may injure yourself. Elite athletes in particular may push through pain that is signaling them to slow down.

The real learning comes in how you handle the aftermath.

Deepening body awareness will help you prevent injury. But another important element in a yoga practice is learning the difference between intensity and pain. In an intense pose, your legs may tremble or you may want to give up. Instead, breathe deeply to build endurance. Sharp, shooting pain, a snap or a pop or feeling like you pulled something, however, indicates it is time to stop.

The first step in assessing your injury is to ask yourself where it bothers you. Pick out the activity where it bothers you, and get down to the details. Does it hurt when I push off my heel, or is it in my knee in a lunge or when I go down the stairs? Does it hurt every time, or only when I move in certain directions? Does it hurt when I'm not moving at all?

If you're really curious, you can go online and find out a common compensation for someone, say, in a lunge with knee pain. You might find out you're not using your butt muscles. If you can stop the compensation, you can come back from the injury once you let the acute injury heal, according to Seattle physical therapist Mark Trombold. If you are uncertain on any level about an injury, go see a professional.

Sometimes you may find that you're not injured, but instead facing a strength deficit. Your body may compensate for a weakness, and that can cause an injury. It will use the strongest muscles rather than the key muscles.

A yoga practice can help you discover your physical weaknesses. When you understand the deficit, you can target particular poses to work on. Once your injury feels better, gradually ease back into activity. Modify your poses or practice as you need to, and spend the time focusing on your breath and listening to your body to know if it's sharp, shooting pain or the shaky intensity that comes with building strength.

THE MENTAL BENEFITS

"Problems are just places where we have been separated from our authentic selves. . . . When you change your focus from limitations to boundless possibilities, from doubt and fear to love and confidence, you open your world in entirely new ways. You stop worrying about fixing what's wrong with you and start living from all that's right within you."

—Baron Baptiste, *Journey into Power*

After her fall, sometimes when Rannveig Aamodt climbed, something would trigger in her. She would freeze, her body paralyzed. She couldn't move. Aamodt would flash back to Turkey in April 2012, the day she tumbled fifty feet to the ground and broke both ankles and her elbow, and fractured her pelvis and three vertebrae. (Learn more about her in her profile below.)

It's natural to be afraid of falling, and climbers constantly face fear. Even before the accident, Aamodt says being comfortable with falling and trusting that her equipment would catch her was a process for her. But after the fall, after the slow excruciating work to get back on her feet, the fear felt different, deeper.

Yoga, a practice she had done for years, helped her to climb again. Before Aamodt could walk again, she did yoga in a chair. Once she could stand, yoga helped her observe unevenness in her body. When she thought about making the return to climbing, yoga helped her tap into her own strength to do just that. And now, if her own body betrays her, she breathes. "Yoga teaches me to take control over my breath," she says. "Even if you're scared, you can at least take control of breath."

Overcoming limitations is built into a climber's bones. When staring up at a 12-pitch climb, you have felt fear of the unknown. You've triple-checked your and your partner's gear, given yourself a little pep talk, and stepped up to the rock. When your arms are pumped and you feel like you can't hang on any longer, you have more than once paused, shaken out your arms, recommitted to your climb, and continued. When you send a boulder problem you once thought impossible,

RANNVEIG AAMODT
Estes Park, Colorado

In 2012, Rannveig Aamodt fell fifty feet. She broke her talus bones in her ankles, her pelvis, her lower back, and one of her elbows. She didn't know if she would climb again. But she wanted to.

While in her hospital bed, she would visualize climbing, the magic of the flow, and how it felt to make her way up a wall. But if she thought about all the steps it would take to walk again, let alone climb, she would tailspin, feeling overwhelmed by all the work it would take to get there. She reminded herself to focus instead on the goal for that day, like touching her nose.

"It would be too much," she said. "Yoga helped me to be present in every day." She did yoga in a chair when she still couldn't use her feet. As she grew stronger, yoga helped her observe unevenness in her body. Slowly, she moved into standing poses.

Aamodt is stronger now and climbs harder routes than she did before the fall. But it took her a long time to feel comfortable climbing—and falling—again. Yoga breathing helped her slow down her breath again, stop sweating, and calm her mind.

She is still surprised sometimes when she gets triggered while climbing—it's unlike anything she experienced before the fall. Aamodt's body freezes; she describes it as "I just stop working." It scares her. Through yoga, breathing is now a tool she knows she can rely on when she needs it.

"Even if I can still get into those situations, it's easier to get out of them," she said. Climbing is so active that she likes yoga as a way to slow down, and she does some yoga every morning to wake her mind and body. Yoga also helps her handle the pressure that comes with being a sponsored climber.

"Yoga helps me to think that I'm good enough anyway," she said. "Even if I'm not the best climber in the world, I have other qualities that can inspire people."

The fall has given her perspective, and helps her prioritize and focus on where she is today rather than thinking about what she has no control over. Like anything, people can make climbing what they want: recreational, fun, or competitive, Aamodt says. Yoga has taught her how she gets to live the way she wants. She can make her own definition of success. "It's helped me to have a healthy view of life," she says.

you have felt triumph surge through your veins. You know what it's like to move beyond your limits.

You also have felt the other end of the spectrum—the days when you feel boxed in by pressure. You doubt you can send the next climb. You feel pressure to climb harder. You have the sense that no matter what you do in climbing or in your life, it will never be good enough. You struggle to focus; you can't shake the sense something is off.

Yoga can give you more than a higher heel hook. It also provides tools to understand the powerful nature of climbing and how to apply it to other areas of your life. Through breath and focus in a yoga practice, you can recall the days you are present, note how you got there, and learn to transfer it to life. In yoga, instead of concentrating on the roughness of rock under your fingertips and navigating the next move, you feel your palms on the floor. You observe without attachment if you feel strong or not. You pay attention to your body's signals. You notice when you feel anxious. You bring your attention inward, and you learn to breathe through tough moments in climbing or in your life.

DISCOVER INNER STRENGTH

Every year, I lead a "40 Days to Personal Revolution" program, designed by my yoga teacher Baron Baptiste. Participants do six days a week of yoga, twice-daily meditation, and focus on nutrition. My studio includes a nutrition challenge for the program, and participants have the option to give up caffeine, alcohol, tobacco, or sugar for the six weeks. You can choose one—or all.

At the end of the program, one participant, Ellen, came up to me. In the first meeting, Ellen told the group she was giving up sugar, but she shared with me she also had secretly pledged to her program buddy she would quit smoking.

Ellen had smoked off and on for twenty-one years. She gave up cigarettes when she was pregnant, but picked it up again once her kids were toddlers. Right before starting the "40 Days" program, she completed a yoga teacher training, smoking all the way through it. She started most days with one cigarette and lit one or two more at night.

At fifty-two, Ellen knew smoking was the source of something amiss in her life. But she couldn't identify it. When she signed up for "40 Days," she knew she had the option to give up smoking, but she was undecided at that first meeting.

One theme in the first meeting is integrity, or keeping your word. I remind the students that they—not I—benefit from staying true to their word to practice yoga and meditation. It's the first moment in years some people have taken steps to prioritize their health and well-being over the needs of their kids, spouses, or careers. No matter how much they may want it, they are often resistant to changing their ingrained habits.

It was during that first meeting that Ellen realized she had to quit smoking, if only to prove to herself she could. A regular yoga practice had already taught her she was physically stronger than she thought. She knew somewhere inside, she was mentally stronger than her cigarette habit.

The first two weeks were hard, she says. She was accustomed to looking forward to her evening cigarette when things got tough at work. The thought of that cigarette helped her hang on during the day. When she struggled, she had to find other ways to feel better. She would go to the bathroom at work and do deep breathing or cry as a release.

Ellen occasionally broke on sugar during the six weeks, and she missed some meditation practices. But she didn't light a cigarette. "It was acknowledging I was strong enough to be without," she told me.

During that period, Ellen realized what she had been stuffing down with cigarettes—her angst over her secure corporate job. She had known for years she was unhappy. Instead of making a change, she smoked. With smoking gone, she realized it was time to do something different. Three months after the end of "40 Days," Ellen gave notice at her job. She's taking a road trip, and she says she'll see what's next.

REDUCE STRESS AND ANXIETY

Yoga and meditation help combat stress and give you more tools to listen to your body and improve your overall health. The majority of Americans live with moderate to high stress, the American Psychological Association (APA) has found. The most common reason people don't do more to manage their stress is they say they are too busy. But estimates claim that seventy-five to ninety percent of all primary care doctor visits are stress-related.

Stress takes an immense toll on your body. Our bodies developed the fight-or-flight response to handle genuine emergencies, like an animal attacking. Even though many people no longer live in a dangerous environment, our bodies still experience the fight-or-flight response in reaction to ordinary challenges, like getting stuck in traffic, meeting a project deadline, or managing our finances, the APA says.

Basically, people spend half the day acting like a bear is chasing them around. Any climber knows that moment of panic on a wall, afraid you can't make the next move, that precipitates a fall. If you don't work through your anxiety, that tough move gets even harder and success becomes less likely. Physically, your adrenal glands flood your body with stress hormones. Your muscles grow tense, your pupils dilate, your sense of smell and hearing heighten, your breathing and heart rate ramp up, and you start to sweat.

React like that every day, and the stress shows up in your body—in tight shoulders, tension in your jaw from grinding your teeth, or an aching in your lower back. The physical focus on strength and mobility in yoga helps you function day to day. But layered underneath those physical benefits are critical practices that lessen stress and anxiety, and help you to move through challenging situations.

A technique as simple as looking at a tree can reduce stress. A frequently cited study published in the journal *Science* in 1984 by environmental psychologist Roger Ulrich, showed that hospital patients had shorter hospital stays, took fewer painkillers, and recovered more quickly overall from surgery when they could see a tree out their window. This study is a literal window into why people often feel more at ease in the wilderness: being outside reduces stress. You can take it to another level by bringing in a mindfulness practice when headed to your next outdoor climb. When you pause to gaze at layers of rock exposed by a steady patient river, or halt in your tracks to spot an eagle soaring overhead, something in your mind and body shifts. You forget about your latest project at work, the bothersome neighbor, or long to-do list. Your mind clears. You are present.

Meditation, its own mindfulness practice, produces a state of restful alertness in your body, according to The Chopra Center, a wellness center founded by Drs. Deepak Chopra and David Simon. When in a state of restful response, your heart rate slows down, your blood pressure normalizes, your breathing calms down, you sweat less, the Chopra Center says. Your body also produces less adrenaline and cortisol, your pituitary gland releases more growth hormone, and your immune function improves. A growing body of evidence suggests the amygdala, the area of the brain responsible for fight-or-flight, shrinks with just eight weeks of mindfulness training.

LEARN TO PAUSE

Studies have suggested yoga can have an effect on the brain similar to that of antidepressants and psychotherapy. One study by Duke University researchers published in *Frontiers in Psychotherapy* showed that yoga plays a role in treating depression, sleep challenges, and even in schizophrenia and attention deficit disorder (ADD). Your quality of life also may improve. Free safety Earl Thomas of the Seattle Seahawks told *Mindful*

magazine a meditation and mindfulness practice has changed the way he looks at the world. "It's an inner thing," he said. "When you're quiet and don't say anything, you start to see the unseen. That's why people need to be observant and listen. When I turned my ears to listening, I improved personally and in everything."

I've seen it happen over and over. Take my student Brian. He came every Saturday to my yoga class, riding his bike no matter the weather and smiling a shy hello each week.

I later learned Brian was an alcoholic. He took up yoga at age thirty-one to help him with his sobriety. Yoga helped him feel better physically—and he can now touch his toes. An old shoulder injury healed, allowing him to throw a baseball again. His sciatica eased up. He met his girlfriend at the studio.

The practice was also a window for him to understand why he smoked pot and drank so much—to numb his anxiety. "I had an incredible amount of tension," he says. "I doused it with alcohol."

Through yoga and breathing, he learned to be with his emotions. After class, his mind no longer raced, looping the same repetitive thoughts. He realized if he was feeling angry or stressed or irritable, he could zoom out of his head, ask himself what was going on, and realize that he didn't have to feel that way. In the early days, he got emotional during final rest. "Yoga in a lot of ways is about observing self and being with challenge, not necessarily trying to make it go away," he says.

Once you use the tools consistently, yoga filters into every layer of life. New possibilities emerge through the practices of presence and listening.

TRANSFORMATION AND CHOICE

Yoga teaches you to observe yourself. Perhaps you're obsessed with climbing as a way of checking out because the wall is the only place you feel grounded, and you don't know how to access those feelings of peace at home. A yoga practice can help you figure that out.

At my first yoga teacher training, I sat across from another trainee and repeated my sob story over and over, crying as I talked: My editors at the newspaper had moved me from my dream job to one I didn't want. I listed all of my misery, including layoffs, departures of dear mentors, an unfruitful job search, and what I considered unreasonable demands at work.

Every time I told her the story, her job was to respond, "Blah blah, blah blah." The idea was to repeat the story until I no longer felt suffering. The first few times she blah-blah'd me, I felt anger through my tears. By the eighth telling, the words started to lose their meaning. By the twelfth, I could recount my tale without feeling intense pain, and I noticed how much drama I'd created about my career. It was only a job.

At the training, I set a goal to leave the paper in a year to teach yoga. When I returned from the training, work felt OK. Nothing changed, on the surface. My responsibilities and requests from my editor didn't change. But I did. I went with the flow. I didn't take it personally when I was assigned a story or my editor gave me feedback. I sometimes worked late on deadline, but unlike before, I didn't get angry or resentful. I even thought cheerily for the next few months that I could teach yoga on the side and be content. And for a few months, I felt good.

But when I was honest with myself, I knew the truth—my best self was not thriving at the newspaper. I wasn't aligned to the work any more. I was practicing contentment (*santosha*), a yoga teaching, but I had not been honest (*satya*), another teaching. I was terrified about giving up health insurance and retirement savings to run a business entirely dependent on one person—me. But those reasonable concerns were holding me back. I had to try a life teaching yoga.

I saved more money, plotted, and stressed constantly. A dear friend and mentor advised me to be less Western and deadline-oriented. "Set an intention," she said. Four months later—a year and four months after saying I would leave the newspaper to teach yoga full-time—I did.

When I wonder what I am supposed to do, who I am supposed to be with, what is next, or why am I here on this planet, I have learned that I must first stop spinning out on my thoughts. Anxiety, fear, and doubt feel heavy in my head, stomach, and face. When I am present, I am excited, energized, and ready for what's next. I let my intuition guide me.

I go to yoga, or I meditate, or I pause in the midst of what I am doing. I see what is true about myself and what I can do. Instead of questioning myself, I have tackled harder climbs than I give myself credit for. Instead of being afraid of the response, I said "I love you" first to my partner. When I wondered if I was certifiably insane each time I quit financially stable jobs to follow a dream, I still did it—first, to teach yoga, and second, to write a book.

Each time that I had fear or doubt, I stopped, listened to my body, identified fear and doubt—and moved forward. When I don't know what is next, I practice. When I am struggling, I practice. When I use the tools consistently, yoga filters into every layer of life. Deep down, the practice of presence may be what drew you to climbing—now, consider how to bring that practice everywhere else.

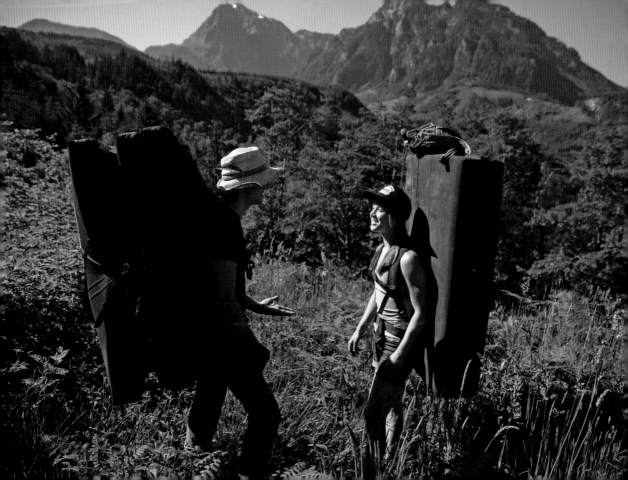

CHAPTER 3
YOGA POSES FOR CLIMBERS

AS A CLIMBER, YOU know strength. You are well practiced on how to execute a power move on a boulder, exploding from your legs and torso to reach for the next hold. You know endurance, climbing pitch after pitch on a tall rock wall to test your body's limits to go ever higher. You know focus, working on the same elusive, next-level route, refining your technique to solve problems that remain just out of reach.

Powerful climbing relies on a foundation of strength. Finger strength allows you to hang onto a crimp hold with just your fingertips. Leg strength helps you balance on one foot while maneuvering to the next hold. Shoulder strength keeps you moving ever upward.

But somewhere along the way, the need for balance shows up. You may notice first that you have a slight hitch in your shoulders or a twinge in your elbow. Or you are frustrated you can't step as high as you'd like because of tight hips. You look at your hands and realize they don't open the way they did before you started climbing.

Physical balance in your body not only prevents injury, it allows you to do sports other than climbing (*gasp*), to know your body more deeply, and to know the full range of your body's capabilities. By focusing on strengthening all the muscles in your shoulders, not just the ones you are accustomed to using to climb, your shoulders will be stronger and more stable. By stretching your feet, you counter the effects of tight climbing shoes and stabilize the muscles that keep you upright while walking. When you understand the mechanics of a twist, you protect your lower back

POSE BASICS

....

Bring your feet together: This is a cue for neutral alignment in your feet. Yoga poses start with feet pointed straight ahead. For most people, it is big toe knuckles touching, with a slight gap at the heels so the outer edges of your feet are roughly parallel to each other.

Four corners of your feet: This refers to your big toe knuckle, pinky toe knuckle, and the two sides of your heels. Balance and your foundation start here by distributing your weight evenly among these four corners of your feet in all poses. If your foot is off the floor, stretch out your toes and continue to activate the four corners.

Core lock: Pull your belly button up and in toward your mid-back to stabilize your spine and trunk.

Hip-width distance: Make fists with your hands, fold forward and place them between your feet to set your feet at hip-width distance. In some cases, like Downward-Facing Dog, you will have to visualize it.

Sit bones: The bones at the base of your pelvis, which you might feel after sitting for a long time on a hard bleacher, are a reference point for alignment. (See figure 4, muscles of the core, in this chapter.)

Pelvic bowl: Your pelvis is shaped like a bowl. Out of habit, most of us stand with it tilting slightly forward or back. Engage your core lock and tilt your tailbone toward the floor to move it into a neutral position. You can bring your hands to your hips to check your pelvic bowl position.

and know how to twist even more gracefully in between moves.

Creating balance starts with noticing what is going on in your body. Understanding how your body functions and seeing ways to counter the effects of climbing ultimately will help you understand your body better and help you access your climbing potential. And if you train off the wall to take on healthy alignment, you will do it subconsciously while climbing.

"Climbers go into [yoga] class with the idea, 'I'll get better range of motion,'" says chiropractor and climber Stephen Sherman. "They can really help their climbing by getting greater control and working on proprioception (understanding of how the body moves in space) of different joints."

Climbing requires endurance, strength, and mental focus; it does plenty to push you physically. Supporting your body, from strengthening to rest, on the days you are not climbing is also vital. A yoga practice is an excellent complement to regular climbing at the gym in winter and outdoors in the summer. Yoga offers physical strengthening, endurance and cardiovascular conditioning. It also provides new tools for staying present and expanding mental stamina on the wall.

Take on a powerful, vinyasa practice once or twice a week, and you may be surprised at your gains, whether it's being less prone to injury, feeling rejuvenated rather than tired and sore the next day, or adding in some ease while taking on the next, tough climb. Add in a weekly restorative practice, and you may be amazed at how relaxed you can feel. Your overall health and mindset can shift more than you know.

This chapter covers major areas of the body that are affected on a climb, from the soles of your feet to your spine. Each section highlights yoga poses that can support a specific area, especially if you

INDIVIDUAL POSES COVERED IN THIS CHAPTER

....

- » Mountain Pose
- » Tree
- » Toes Pose
- » Halfway Lift
- » Crescent Lunge
- » Half Pigeon
- » Side Plank
- » Reverse Tabletop
- » Eagle
- » Downward-Facing Dog
- » Plank
- » Seated Twist
- » Locust

are prone to injury. Please note that this is meant to be a glimpse into the poses and that they are most beneficial when included in a full practice with a warm-up and cool down. All poses in this chapter are included in the Strength and Recovery practices that offer a full practice.

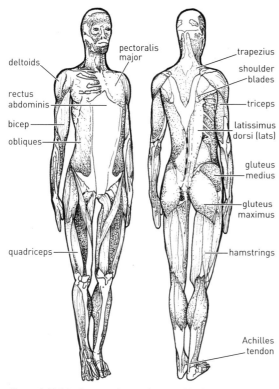

deltoids

pectoralis
major

rectus
abdominis

bicep

obliques

quadriceps

trapezius

shoulder
blades

triceps

latissimus
dorsi (lats)

gluteus
medius

gluteus
maximus

hamstrings

Achilles
tendon

Figure 1. Full body musculature, front and back

SUPPORT YOUR FEET

Trusting your feet is one of the first techniques climbers learn. Even if you feel you've mastered this important body part, spending time focusing on your feet will improve your climbing foundation.

Your feet bear your weight throughout a climb, and are the foundation for your time on the wall. Your feet have twenty-eight bones each, with four layers of musculature, a bottom layer called your plantar fascia (see figure 2), and the pads of your feet. When the bones and muscles work together, they create lift, balance, and movement in your foot, according to well-known anatomy expert Leslie Kaminoff in *Yoga Anatomy*. Feet adapt incredibly well to uneven terrain, critical to staying balanced on just your big toe on a tiny hold. But most people spend the majority of time on smooth, artificially even surfaces common in our modern world. Over time, if they are not challenged, the deeper muscles that support your feet weaken and only the surface layer, the plantar fascia, prevent collapse.

A climbing wall continually challenges the musculature of your feet, but the constant pressure on the inside of your big toe—in addition

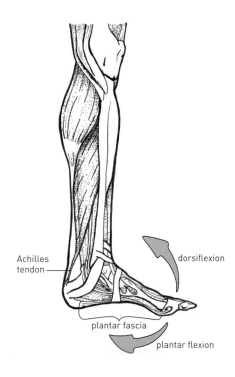

Achilles
tendon

dorsiflexion

plantar fascia

plantar flexion

Figure 2. Muscles of the feet and ankles

to cramped climbing shoes that squish your big toe—means the muscles mainly work in one direction. By doing yoga poses in bare feet, stretching the big toe muscle in the opposite direction and practicing balancing your weight evenly over the sole of your foot, you condition your feet to maintain strength, balance, and integrity.

POSES FOR FEET

Mountain Pose

A foundational pose for the entire practice, Mountain Pose starts with awareness in your feet. It engages your whole foot and creates strength. The pose also illuminates weaknesses in your feet, allowing you to work that area.

» Stand with your feet directly underneath your hips with the outer edges of your feet parallel to your mat, arms relaxed by your sides.
» Lift and spread your toes, creating gaps between every toe from your big toe to your pinky toe. Notice how this lifts the arches of your feet.
» Soften your toes to the floor. Press the four corners of your feet into the floor.

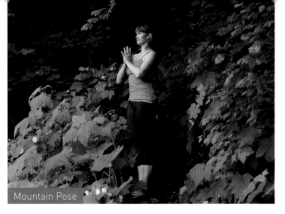

Mountain Pose

» Keep your feet grounded and spin your inner ankles toward the back of your mat. Energetically draw your outer ankles down toward the floor.

» Fold forward toward your shins. Cross your wrists, palms facing away from each other, and bring your palms to your inner calves. Press opposite palms into opposite inner calves. Notice the action in your feet, calves, and inner thighs.

» Stand up slowly. Keep your awareness in your feet. Close your eyes and notice how your feet flex and balance to keep your body upright.

Tree

A simple balancing pose, Tree focuses attention on your feet and ankles to engage micro-stabilizing muscles, which develops stability and strength. Your inner thigh muscles lengthen and your rear muscles engage. You also will open your hip on your lifted leg.

» Stand with your feet together. Feel the four corners of your feet on the floor or mat.

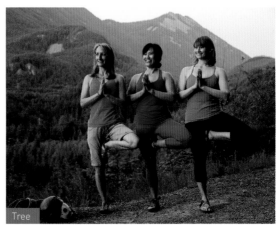

Tree

» Lift one foot to either your inner calf, or above your knee joint to your inner thigh. If balancing is challenging, prop the foot of your bent leg against the ankle of your standing foot with the ball of your foot on the floor.
» Pull your belly in toward your spine to engage your core.
» Bring your palms together at the center of your chest. Stay for five breaths.

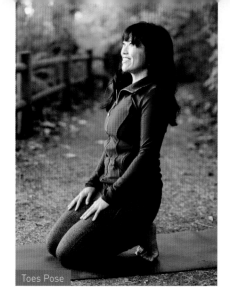
Toes Pose

Toes Pose

Many people find this pose quite intense. Toes Pose opens your toes, and stretches both your Achilles tendon and the fascia in the soles of your feet. You may not have stretched your ankles and feet in this direction before. Work up toward holding this pose. You can modify Toes Pose by tucking a rolled-up blanket behind your knees. Do not stay in the pose if it is painful for you.

» Come to your knees on a mat. Tuck your toes underneath you until you are on the balls of your feet—tuck your pinky toes in if they escape.
» Sit up slowly and lift your chest over your hips until you feel the sensation in your feet.

» Breathe deeply for thirty seconds, or stay up to one minute.
» Counter pose: Shift forward onto your hands and knees. Release your toe tuck and point your toes on the floor. Bring your hands to the ground behind you and lean back on your feet to stretch into your shins, the front of your foot and your ankles in the opposite direction to counter the intensity.

RELEASE YOUR HIPS AND GLUTES

Unlock your hips and you are on the road to access your full potential on a climb. You may already know tight hips prevent you from reaching distant holds on a route you have zeroed in on. The more you open your hips, the easier it will be to get a higher heel hook. Understanding how your hips rotate also will give you a new perspective on how to adjust your body next to the wall while climbing. Learning to hinge at your hips with a long flat back in a Halfway Lift will help strengthen your lower back and teach your body to rely on bigger, stronger muscles in your hips. Strengthening your glutes and other muscles around your hips also will give you more power on the wall.

Your pelvis grounds and stabilizes your body. You use the muscles attached to your pelvis daily, relying on the psoas muscle deep in your hip to get out of bed. Your gluteus maximus and gluteus medius, the big butt muscles, and hamstrings kick in when you walk. (See figure 3, muscles of the hips, glutes, and hamstrings.) And yet most people don't know how to engage their glutes. Weak glutes, a result of sitting and general

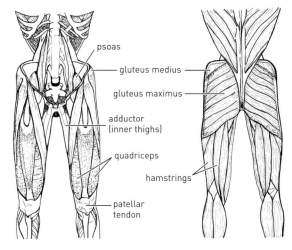

Figure 3. Muscles of the hips, glutes, and hamstrings

underuse, can lead you to overrely on your lower back when walking or twisting. Your hip flexors also get shorter from sitting at a 90-degree angle all day.

Your pelvis has big flat bones with lots of muscles attached. It's easy for tension to get locked up in your hips, buried among all those muscles and connectors, and it takes time to release. Tension in your hips often works its way into your lower back, and stretching your hips also can provide some release from lower back pain. Rather than focusing solely on hip rotation for climbing, be mindful of the burden your hips and glutes take on every day to keep you moving. Hip-release poses help your muscles relax and let go, while strengthening your glutes will provide more durability when you need the endurance.

POSES FOR HIPS AND GLUTES

Halfway Lift

Essentially a hip hinge, Halfway Lift builds upon Mountain Pose and challenges you to engage your core, activate your hamstrings, and strengthen your lower back. It also teaches your body to bend at the hips versus at your lower back. (See photo on p. 101.)

» Bring your big toes to touch. Stretch your toes and connect the four corners of your feet to the floor.

» Place your hands on your shins. Bend your knees and squeeze your thighs.
» Lengthen your chest parallel to the floor. Stretch your sit bones toward to the wall behind you and spin them out from each other.
» Hug your shoulder blades onto your spine and stretch your chest longer.
» Lift your head in line with your spine. Set your gaze past the top of your mat.
» Stay for ten rounds of breath.

Crescent Lunge

Holding Crescent Lunge for a long time tests your balance, stabilizes your knees and ankles, and teaches you to breathe through challenge! Your hips internally rotate to stabilize in Crescent Lunge, and by pulling your thigh bones into your pelvis, you can practice pulling into a strong, stable centerline.

» Step into a long lunge with right foot forward, left foot back. Stack your right knee over the ankle of your right foot. Lift your left heel so your toes are bent and the sole of your foot is

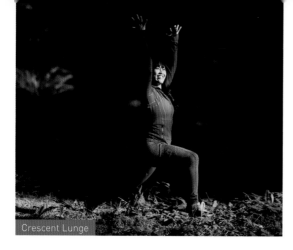

Crescent Lunge

» To intensify, lower your back knee so it hovers two inches from the ground. Hold for five breaths. Straighten your back leg. Switch sides.

Half Pigeon

As much as you need to strengthen your hips, it is important to relax the muscles that support your pelvis. Half Pigeon is a restorative pose that works in your hip to release your piriformis, a hip stabilizer, and also releases in your butt muscles. Your front leg rotates out, and it will work deeply into the muscles around your hips. If you climb outdoors frequently, hip release also is important to soften from the intensity of additional weight your lower body bears from carrying heavy ropes, carabiners, and other gear.

» From a seated position, bend your right leg in front of you. Move your right thigh parallel to the outer edge of your mat with your right foot tucked in toward your pelvis. Flex your right foot to protect your knee.

» Extend your left leg straight behind you so that the top of your thigh is on the ground.

perpendicular to the ground. Move your feet hip-width distance apart for stability.

» Lift your chest over your hips and extend your arms up to the ceiling.

» Squeeze your back hamstring straight.

» Pull your belly in and up to support your core.

» Square your pelvis toward the front of your mat.

» Reach your arms up parallel to your ears, pinky fingers forward.

» Stay for five breaths, then switch sides.

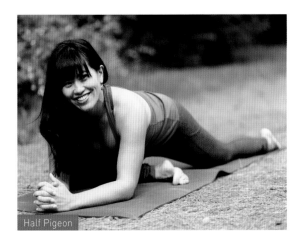
Half Pigeon

» Flex your toes on your back foot and come up to the ball of your foot.
» Roll up to center so your pelvis is squared toward the front of your mat. Place a block under your right hip if you have trouble staying centered.
» Lengthen your chest and lower your torso toward the floor. Stay here for twenty breaths. Switch sides.

» Deepen: If you don't feel sensation in your hip, move your front shin toward parallel with the front edge of your mat.
» Modify: If you have knee injuries and this pose exacerbates any pain in your knees, take a Reclined Half Pigeon. (See p. 126 in Strength Practice I in chapter 4.)

TIGHTEN YOUR CORE

Your trunk holds you up—and together! Taking care of it will keep your body healthy long-term. Think of it like a canister, says chiropractor and climber Stephen Sherman, with a base of your pelvic floor, a top with your diaphragm, and muscles that make up the circular sides, including your abdominals, side oblique muscles, the tiny muscles of your spine, and more.

Using your diaphragm is a key step to understanding your core. In a yoga practice, ujjayi breathing teaches you to move your diaphragm for your breath and engage your belly muscles. People with shoulder injuries in particular can use their shoulders and other muscles to breathe, Sherman says. Engaging the diaphragm to support the core

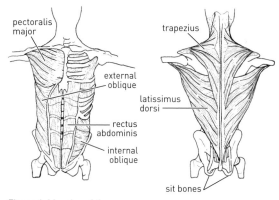

Figure 4. Muscles of the core

in backbends. Your obliques along the side of your trunk contribute to twisting, while the transverse addominus, the deepest abdominal muscle, supports *uddhiyana bandha*. Your back and shoulder muscles connect into your glutes, so the stronger you keep your back muscles overall, the stronger you will feel in your lower body.

Endurance also is an important element to core stability. Once you build your core strength, it will be natural for you to engage it when you climb—your technique will flow naturally from your center.

POSE FOR YOUR CORE

Side Plank

Side Plank challenges your external oblique muscles in your torso as well as other parts of your core. It works deep into your glutes and the lower arm and shoulder holding you up, firing the muscles on half of your body. It also strengthens your hands and wrists. The goal is for your body to stabilize using neutral alignment of your spine and legs.

» Plant your hands under your shoulders for Plank. Tuck your toes and lift your knees off

and stop using unnecessary muscles for a basic function is job one.

The core lock used in yoga also teaches you to tilt your pelvis to a neutral position. Your pelvis is shaped like a bowl, and you want it to be level, tipping neither forward nor backward. Your core lock also engages multiple levels of muscles that support your spine, including your rectus abdominis, the central washboard muscles seen on some and used by all, that play a role in Forward Folds and protects the lower spine (lumbar)

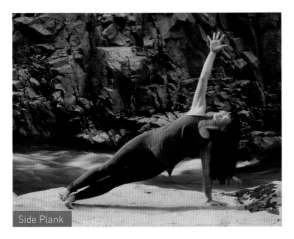
Side Plank

the ground. Bring your hips slightly below level with your shoulders.

» From Plank, bring your feet to touch. Roll onto the outer edge of your right foot with your left foot stacked on top.

» Stack your right shoulder over your right wrist; all your weight will be on your right hand. Your right hand faces the front of the mat and is stacked just a couple of inches forward of your shoulder.

» Lift your left hand up to the ceiling, palm facing the same direction as your chest.

» Flex your toes toward your knees and squeeze the muscles of your legs to the bone.

» Keep your body at one angled plane from shoulders to feet.

» Set your gaze and look up to the ceiling.

» Stay for ten breaths. Switch to your left hand.

» Modify: Bring your lower knee to the floor and stack it under your hip. Keep your lower hand, knee, and foot in line with each other. Use your core to stabilize in the pose.

OPEN YOUR SHOULDERS AND ELBOWS

Your upper body is taxed on the wall as it continually pulls you upward hold by hold. Your shoulders in particular take on a heavy load as you climb. Athletes who reach overhead generally need some mobility in their mid-back, the thoracic spine, but since most people spend their days slumped forward, their shoulders a casualty of gravity, the spine locks up fairly easily. If you don't focus on rotating your mid-spine, you most likely compensate by reaching through your lower back or your

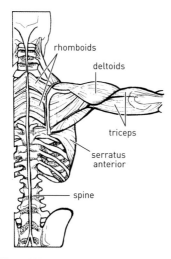

Figure 5. Muscles of the spine and shoulders

shoulders for strength. If you are suffering from a lot of shoulder and elbow injuries, consider it a signal that you lack balance in your upper body. Your back is packed with powerful, strong muscles, and when you instead rotate your shoulders back toward your spine and access the multiple layers of muscles in your core, you will have more strength and endurance overall, not to mention happier, healthier shoulders.

Training your shoulders to rotate toward your back to open your chest will create balance in your shoulder strength and also lengthen your spine. Pulling your upper arm bones into your shoulder sockets and adding weight, like a plank, will get your body accustomed to engaging new muscles for a healthier shoulder girdle.

Another common shoulder challenge is shoulder impingement. Think of a belayer, shoulders slumped forward with chin jutted forward and his head tilted back looking up at the climber. In this position, the rotator cuff or the bicep tendon can get pinched from the constant roll forward.

When focusing on your shoulders, soften your trapezius, the muscles under your ears, and pull your shoulder blades in toward your spine.

neck, forcing your shoulder to do more work than it needs to, says Sherman.

In climbing, people tend to bend their elbows and rotate their shoulders forward toward their chest, relying on their chest and the front of their

Activate the muscles underneath your shoulder blades and the serratus anterior, which wrap around your ribs. By activating different muscles, you'll learn to externally rotate and protect your shoulders while you climb. Backbends are an important practice to rotate your shoulders externally and open tight chest muscles.

Shoulder health is a priority for any climber. If you take good care of your shoulders, your elbows will by extension be healthier, and your climbing will get stronger.

COMMON INJURIES

» Elbow tendinitis: If tendons get injured and you keep climbing, your elbow tendons will degenerate over time.
» Tennis (or golfer's) elbow: With so much time spent gripping holds, the flexors in your hands work more than the extensors that straighten your hands, and that imbalance can move into your elbow causing pain at the joint.
» Shoulder impingement: When your shoulders are constantly internally rotated, your rotator cuff or bicep tendon can get pinched, causing pain in the shoulder.

POSES FOR SHOULDERS AND ELBOWS

Reverse Tabletop

Reverse Tabletop is a modified backbend that deeply stretches your pectoral muscles, your deltoids, and your biceps opening your chest, shoulders, and upper arms. It reverses the feeling of gravity pulling forward on your shoulders. Your triceps straighten your arms.

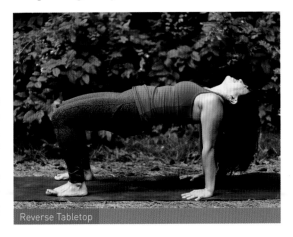

Reverse Tabletop

» From a seated position, place your hands behind you with your fingertips facing your body.
» Walk your feet in toward you so they are flat on the floor at hip-width distance.
» Ground into the four corners of your feet, and lift your hips toward the ceiling.
» Press your palms into the ground.
» Lengthen the crown of your head behind you. Gently release your head onto your shoulders.
» Stay for five breaths.

Eagle

Eagle challenges your balance and the bind opens your shoulders. Be patient if you can't immediately bind and try the modification for now. Your shoulders will open over time.

» Stand in Mountain Pose. Reach your arms out parallel to the floor, palms facing forward. Cross your right upper arm under your left upper arm. Wind your forearms around each other. Bring your palms to touch for the full bind.
» Lift your elbows even with your shoulders. Press your hands away from your face to vertical so your wrists stack over your elbows.

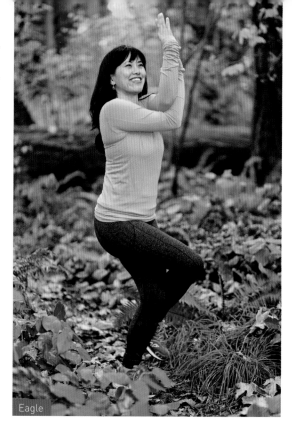
Eagle

» With your big toes touching, bend your knees to lower your hips toward the floor for Chair. Cross your right thigh on top of your left thigh. Your upper foot can dangle; stretch out your toes to activate your foot. Squeeze your inner thighs.
» Stay for five breaths. Switch sides.
» Modify: If you can't wrap your arms for the full bind, take hold of opposite shoulders. Lift your elbows off your chest.

BALANCE YOUR HANDS AND WRISTS

When you first learned to climb, you probably realized rather quickly that it requires strong hands and wrists. Over time, your hands may have gotten so strong and accustomed to a curled position for holds, that the flexors are now stronger than the extensors that straighten your fingers, which can lead to tendinitis. Balancing out the strength in your hands will in turn keep your wrists healthy.

In addition to stretching, focus on strengthening your hands and wrists in the opposite direction of climbing. Yoga poses like Downward-Facing Dog are an excellent place to practice both.

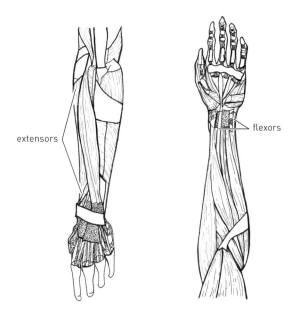

extensors

flexors

Figure 6. Muscles of the forearms and wrists

Downward-Facing Dog

Downward-Facing Dog is a widely used pose for good reason—it has benefits for the whole body. An inverted V-shape, it lengthens your hamstrings, your calves, and your spine, and in the pose, you practice grounding into your hands and learning to open and strengthen your shoulders. This pose is a good place to pay attention to your sit bones, the bones at the base of your pelvis. (See figure 4, muscles of the core.) In Downward-Facing Dog, practice spinning your sit bones up to the ceiling to lengthen your spine and engage your core.

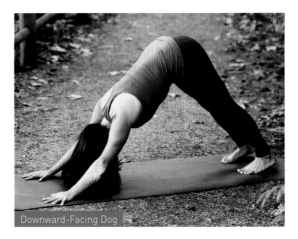
Downward-Facing Dog

» Come to your hands and knees, with your hands positioned underneath your shoulders, index finger pointing straight forward.
» Tuck your toes underneath you, and lift your hips up to the ceiling. Walk your feet back about six inches.
» Bend your knees and lift your tailbone until your spine lengthens. Spin your sit bones to the wall behind you.
» Roll your shoulders up to your ears, then use your back muscles to pull your shoulders down and in toward your spine. Squeeze your upper arms toward each other.
» Drive your heels toward the floor (they don't need to touch the floor).
» Pull your belly in toward your spine.
» Lift the muscles just above your knees to engage your thighs and open into your hamstrings. Stay for fifteen full breaths.

Plank

Plank pose is commonly used as a core strengthener. In yoga, the emphasis on doing a Plank on your hands rather than elbows brings awareness to your palms as your foundation and strengthens your wrists by pushing into the floor. Flatten your hands onto the floor and stretch your fingers out to counter any clenching from climbing. This is also a good place to work on rotating your shoulders down your back and strengthening your shoulders. If that wasn't enough, Plank also strengthens your thighs and the oblique muscles along the lateral sides of your torso.

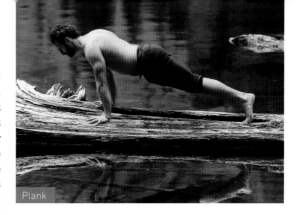
Plank

» Come to your hands and knees on your mat. Stack your hands underneath your shoulders, index finger pointed straight ahead.
» Step your feet to the back of your mat. Tuck your toes and lift your knees off the floor, and squeeze your legs straight.
» Keep your hips just below level with your shoulders.
» Lift your head so your neck is level with your shoulders.

» Spiral your inner thighs up to the ceiling. Lengthen the backs of your knees and squeeze your thighs. Tilt your tailbone toward your heels.
» Press your palms firmly into the floor. Squeeze your upper arm bones toward each other.
» Spin the inner eye of your elbows forward, and pull your shoulder blades together.
» Lift your belly in toward your spine and wrap your front ribs together.
» Breathe and hold for one minute. If you can't hold for one minute, build up to it. Repeat three times.

» To modify the pose, bring your knees to the floor. Keep your hips on an even plane between your shoulders and your knees, belly muscles fully engaged.

TWIST AND LENGTHEN YOUR SPINE AND NECK

Your spine is the central pillar of your body, and you want to keep it supple and strong. Adding in twists to rotate your spine keeps it flexible by encouraging the muscles between vertebrae and around your spine to open up. Backbends strengthen the muscles that arch your back and keep your spine in healthy alignment.

If height is not on your side in climbing, take comfort in knowing that if you work on lengthening your spine through twists and backbends, you can get added extension to grab a hold that looks out of reach. Twists and backbends develop more body awareness around your spine, and you will learn to reach from your spine rather than your shoulders. By using the following poses to understand what it feels like to extend while you're still safely on the ground, it will become natural when you're reaching for holds on a massive rock face.

POSES FOR SPINE AND NECK

Seated Twist

A simple twist you can do anywhere, Seated Twist will offer release from long periods of sitting or from a big day outside.

» From a seated position, extend your right leg straight to the front of your mat, toes flexed. Bend your left knee and walk your left foot in close to your hip.

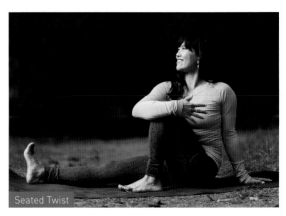

Seated Twist

» Place your left hand on the floor behind you. Reach your right arm up to the ceiling, then wrap it around your bent leg.
» Stay for ten breaths. Switch sides.

Locust

Backbends build strength in your spine and also work deeply into the big back muscles in your torso that support your spine. Locust pose focuses on the muscles that arch the back and is helpful for strengthening your lower back.
» Lie on your belly. Bring your feet to hip-width distance, toes pointed.
» Reach your hands alongside your body, hands down by your hips, palms facing down.
» Pull your belly in toward your spine.

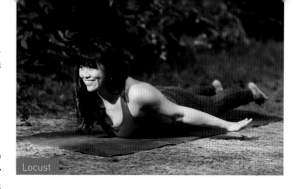

Locust

» Press the tops of your feet into the floor, and lift your knees off the ground. Keep your upper legs engaged, and lift them off the floor.
» Lift your upper arm bones toward the ceiling and float your hands above your hips.
» Set your gaze on a point on the ground below your nose. Stay for ten breaths.

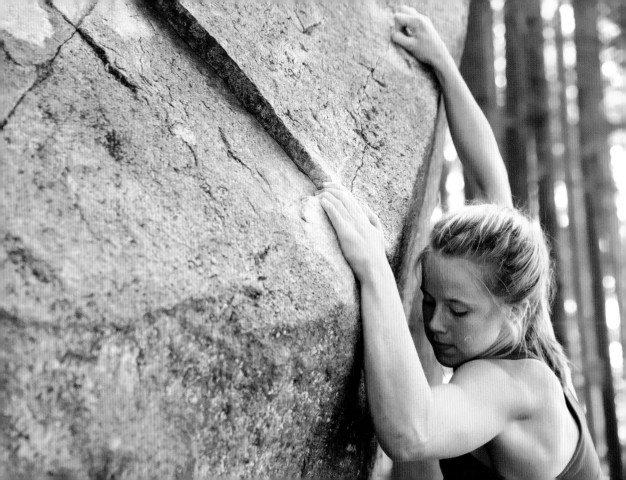

CHAPTER 4
YOGA PRACTICES FOR CLIMBERS

I OFTEN REMIND STUDENTS when they get perfectionistic about yoga poses to remember it is called a yoga *practice*. The power comes from doing it over and over. When you put your body into different shapes that challenge your strength and flexibility, pay attention to alignment, and meld poses with breath, it is a formidable combination. The more you practice and pay attention to your body in poses, the more you rewire your body and your mind. And that repeated effort gives you access to the subterranean levels of change and growth available in a yoga practice.

In this chapter, you will learn about a power yoga practice. Physical power in your body can be interpreted as bursts of speed, like a power move to reach for a hold. In yoga, power stems from

holding poses to build stability, building heat in your body from those holds, and experiencing freedom physically through alignment.

You will encounter challenge—that is a major component of your yoga practice. Rather than muscling through or forcing your body, consider breathing more deeply, listening and seeing if you can shift your alignment or your perspective in a pose you initially find tough. Take Child's Pose to return to your intentional ujjayi breath.

The sequences in this chapter are designed for two different approaches—strength and recovery. The Strength Practices will support you while climbing, creating stability and endurance in your lower body, spine, and core as well as dynamically opening into your hips and shoulders. The later sequences include poses to practice before you climb and at the end of a long day climbing to support your body to stay at its most optimal.

In the Strength Practices, you will do poses to connect to your body so that you can let go mentally. Strength Practice I will build your strength in a short amount of time. Your heart rate will elevate and you will sweat! Do it regularly to get stronger and practice noticing your body sensations. In Strength Practice II you will build upon what you learned in the first, adding on more challenging poses and pushing your endurance for a longer stretch of time. Both practices start by activating your core, then move you into Sun Salutations, which are a traditional way to open a vinyasa practice. They build heat through repetition and help you practice connecting breath with movement. Once your body becomes accustomed to opening your practice this way, you will notice more ease and flow.

The standing poses for both practices build stability, challenge balance, and open your spine. They are strong poses designed to push you to your edge. The balancing poses strengthen your feet and test your body's limits to keep you upright, while arm balances test your skills and determination! Keep going.

Backbends open your chest and heart. Most of us habitually hunch forward, our posture sloppy from years of slouching. Backbends require us to reverse those years of habit, and they are a particularly effective way for climbers to stretch the muscles in the chest and practice external shoulder rotation. You may feel some resistance to backbends when first starting, partly because of your body's physical ways, and also the energetic opening experience that comes with a backbend. It can feel uncomfortable to release in your chest and around your heart if you are not used to it. Be patient and soften in your chest. You never know what you may find.

Inversions turn your perspective upside down. Seeing your legs in the air may be all it takes. When your body is upside down, more blood moves to your heart, pumping more efficiently and slowing your heart rate and your blood pressure. Your heart gets a break and in turn, you relax.

You may be tempted to skip Final Rest. Savor it. It's the key to letting all the energy you've opened up in your body resettle. It trains you to restore. It offers a space of stillness—all too rare in a busy day.

All the practices include recovery poses, particularly important for athletes who push their limits day in and day out. If you normally take a rest day after a long day climbing, do the Recovery Practice. It is designed for a body that feels achy and tired. Your muscles and energy contract after a lot of intensity, and the recovery sequence will allow your body to both open and heal from a big day outdoors.

These practices are intended to support your time climbing both at the gym and outdoors, and a regular practice is key to seeing a shift. To experience the most impact physically and mentally, do one Strength Practice at least twice a week, but know that it is designed to practice daily. Build from the 25-minute sequence to the 45-minute one. Do the Recovery Practice once a week.

"Practice, practice, practice. That's it."

—Sri K Pattabhi Jois, in an interview

UNDERSTANDING THE POSES

Each pose description includes the following:
» **Name:** Common English name for the pose.
» **Introduction:** Context for the pose, relationship to the body, and how the pose supports you on the rock.
» **Setup:** Getting into the pose.
» **Alignment:** Specific cues to pay attention to for proper body alignment.
» **Release:** Some poses have directions for a specific release.
» **Gaze & focus:** Where to set your drishti (gaze) during the pose and where to focus your attention within your body during a pose.
» **Deepen:** Ways to deepen a pose for the next level of challenge.
» **Common challenges:** Physical challenges you may experience during the pose.
» **Modifications:** Alternatives to modify the full pose.

For poses that are already modifications of the full pose, challenges and modifications are not listed.

SEQUENCE FOR STRENGTH PRACTICE I

» Supine Butterfly
» Happy Baby
» Boat
» Plank
» Low Cobra
» Child's Pose
» Downward-Facing Dog

» Rag Doll
» Halfway Lift
» Mountain Pose
» Sun Salutation A
» Sun Salutation B
» Gorilla
» Twisted Chair
» Low Lunge

» Twisted Crescent Lunge
» Warrior 2
» Triangle
» Side Angle
» Eagle
» Tree
» Flip Dog

» Side Plank
» Bow
» Bridge
» Reclined Half Pigeon
» Seated Forward Fold
» Seated Twist
» Legs Up the Wall
» Corpse Pose

GET READY

The Strength Practices are based on a power vinyasa practice. This weaves held poses for stability and challenge with a flow connecting breath and poses to build heat. They are designed to be challenging. You'll find as you grow in strength and mobility, you will build endurance and cultivate ease in the flow. If you start to lose your breath or need a rest at any time, remember you can take Child's pose. Return to your ujjayi breath and then resume the sequence when you are ready.

KEY

Many of the cues are based in Mountain Pose. It is the foundation for your entire practice! The cues for poses also presume you are practicing in a room with walls and a ceiling, but feel free to interpret the cues if you are practicing outdoors. Please note that you have seen some of these poses in chapter 3. For those poses, you will see some additional alignment cues in this chapter to support a deeper understanding and experience of the pose.

Each pose should be held for five full breaths (each breath is made up of both an inhale and an exhale) unless otherwise noted. If there is a necessary transition between poses, you'll see a notation for a Sequence Transition.

STRENGTH PRACTICE I

TIME: 25 MINUTES
EQUIPMENT: YOGA MAT, BLOCK, AND STRAP

RELEASE AND ACTIVATE

This first phase of the sequence is a time to focus on your breath and your core, and in the process, release mental lists. Bring your attention to your physical body and notice your ability to listen to it and learn.

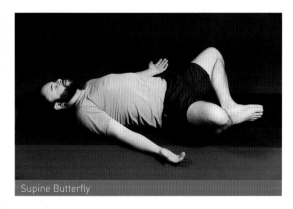
Supine Butterfly

Supine Butterfly

Starting your yoga practice lying on your back gives your body time to relax; the contact between your spine and the floor signals your brain that it's time to let go. Gravity draws your legs down toward the floor, naturally opening your hips. Your shoulders relax down into your mat; close your eyes if you like. Give yourself time in this pose to feel the floor under you and to let your mind settle. Focus on your active ujjayi breath.

SETUP Lay down with your back on your mat.
• Bring the soles of your feet together so your legs form a diamond shape.

ALIGNMENT Let your arms relax on the floor, palms facing up. • Notice the connection of your spine to the floor and the natural curve of your lumbar spine at your lower back. • Hug your belly in and up toward your spine to activate your core. • Bring in your ujjayi breath.

GAZE & FOCUS Close your eyes. • Bring your attention to your spine on the floor and an active core.

COMMON CHALLENGES Tight hips or lower back pain prevent you from relaxing your knees toward the floor.

MODIFICATION Bring your feet as wide as your mat and rest your knees together to bring your lower back to the mat.

Happy Baby

Happy Baby opens your hips and brings your spine into neutral alignment. This is a wonderful pose to check in at the beginning of practice and again at the end to see what has changed in your spine and hips. If you can roll around on the floor and embody the name of this pose, you'll love the pose even more.

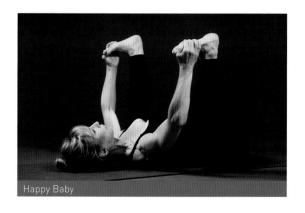
Happy Baby

SETUP From Supine Butterfly, pull your knees into your chest. Take your knees wide outside your chest. • Reach inside your legs for the inner arches of your feet and lift your feet toward the ceiling.

ALIGNMENT Flex your feet toward your knees. Bend your knees at 90 degrees. Press your heels toward the ceiling. • Relax your shoulders. • Lengthen your lower back toward the floor while pulling on your feet with your hands. Press your feet into your hands.

GAZE & FOCUS Look at a spot on the ceiling.
• Lengthen your spine to the mat.

DEEPEN Switch your grip on your feet to the outside arch of your foot; pull your knees deeper down outside your ribs.

COMMON CHALLENGES Tight hips or lower back prevent you from reaching your feet.

MODIFICATION Hold the backs of your thighs instead of your feet. Open your knees wider than your chest.
• Place a block under your head.

SEQUENCE TRANSITION From Happy Baby, pull your knees into your chest. • With momentum, rock up to a seated position.

Boat

You use your core intensely during a climb, and the more you connect to the strength of your trunk, the more you will flow on the wall. One of the most effective ways to strengthen your core,

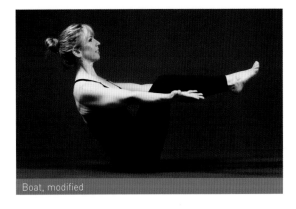
Boat, modified

Boat pose challenges your trunk muscles in multiple ways. That said, people love to cheat this pose! Be sure to lift your chest to get the full impact.

SETUP Hold the backs of your thighs, and balance between your sit bones at the base of your pelvis and your tailbone. Lift your feet off the floor.

ALIGNMENT Pull your thighs toward your chest. Hold your shins parallel to the floor. • Squeeze your thighs toward each other. Spread out your toes so you see a gap between each one. • Pull your shoulder blades toward each other. Lift your chest toward the ceiling. • Reach your arms straight in front of you. • Stay for ten breaths. • Transition to Low Boat pose. Lower until your lower back is on the floor, your shoulders off the floor and your legs hover above the mat. Squeeze your thighs together. Stay for five rounds of breath. • Lift back to Boat. Stay for ten breaths.

GAZE & FOCUS Set your gaze on your toes. • Concentrate on lifting your chest and lengthening your spine.

DEEPEN Once your hamstrings allow it, straighten your legs at a 45-degree angle away from the floor.

COMMON CHALLENGES Lower back weakness prevents you from lifting your chest.

MODIFICATION Hold the back of your thighs to keep your chest lifted.

SEQUENCE TRANSITION From Boat, set your feet on the floor. • Hug your knees and lift your chest to the ceiling to release in your core. • From a seated position, roll over your feet hands and knees. • Plant your hands at the front of your mat and step your feet to the back edge of your mat.

Plank

Your core is the key link for your entire body, and Plank is an effective way to build trunk strength and heat! Plank is also an excellent place to practice Mountain Pose on a different plane, by keeping your legs fully engaged, pulling your shoulder blades into your spine, and lifting your head to be level with the rest of your spine.

SETUP Stack your hands underneath your shoulders, index finger pointed straight ahead. Stay on the balls of your feet, lift your knees off the floor, and squeeze your legs straight.

ALIGNMENT Keep your hips just below level with your shoulders. • Spiral your inner thighs up to the ceiling. Lengthen the backs of your knees and

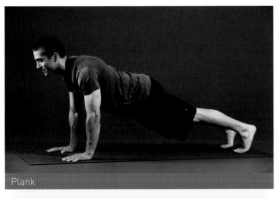

Plank

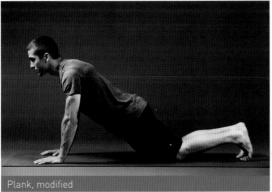

Plank, modified

squeeze your thighs. • Lift your head so your neck is level with your shoulders. • Press your palms firmly into the floor. Squeeze your upper arm bones toward each other. • Spin the inner eye of your elbows forward, and pull your shoulder blades together. • Tilt your tailbone toward your heels. • Lift your belly in toward your spine and wrap your front ribs together. • Stay for ten breaths.

GAZE & FOCUS Set your gaze past the front of your mat. • Keep your legs and core firm. Breathe deeply to maintain the pose.

COMMON CHALLENGES Building strength to hold the full pose for ten breaths can take some practice.

MODIFICATION Bring your knees to the floor, toes curled under. Keep your hips in one line with your shoulders with your core engaged.

SEQUENCE TRANSITION From Plank, shift to the tips of your toes and slowly lower to the floor, chest and pelvis touching down at the same time on the mat.

Low Cobra

A gentle backbend, Low Cobra still has plenty of impact. When practiced diligently with strong legs and a lift in your chest and spine, it builds strength in your back and opens your chest, reversing any forward slump you may have created.

SETUP Press the tops of your toes into the floor. • Squeeze your thighs and lift your knees off the mat. • Place your hands next to your lower ribs so your elbows are at a 90-degree angle.

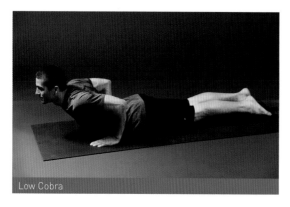

Low Cobra

ALIGNMENT Press your pelvis into the floor. • Engage your core and lift your chest off the floor. Hug your arm bones toward your spine. • Tilt your tailbone toward your heels slightly. • Lift your hands an inch off the floor to take weight out of your hands.

GAZE & FOCUS Lift your gaze forward about a foot in front of you. • Maintain strong legs and lift from your core.

DEEPEN Press your palms down and lift to Upward-Facing Dog (see Strength Practice II).

SEQUENCE TRANSITION Lower your chest back to the floor. • Press up to hands and knees.

Child's Pose

In a world of constant stimulation, Child's Pose offers a quiet, internal space. It brings your focus inward to your body and your breath, and it relaxes your spine and lower back, your hips and your shoulders. This pose is optional; if you would like

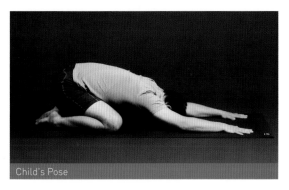
Child's Pose

to skip it, feel free. But remember you can come into this pose any time the practice becomes too intense. Use it to pause and return to your ujjayi breath.

SETUP From hands and knees, bring your big toes together and move your knees to the edges of your mat. Sink your hips back over your heels. Walk your hands forward at shoulder-width distance and bring your forehead to the ground.

ALIGNMENT Let go of tension in your shoulders.
• Engage your core gently, pulling your belly up and in toward your spine. • Come into your ujjayi breath. • Stay for ten breaths.

GAZE & FOCUS Close your eyes. • Deepen your ujjayi breath. Pay attention to the feeling of the mat under your hands and forehead.

COMMON CHALLENGES A tight lower back or hips can prevent your forehead from touching the ground. • Knee injuries can prevent you from bending your knees comfortably.

MODIFICATIONS Bring a block under your forehead to relax your neck. • Roll over onto your back for Supine Butterfly or lay flat on your belly.

SEQUENCE TRANSITION Come up to hands and knees.

Downward-Facing Dog

New students are often skeptical that Downward-Facing Dog can become a resting pose, but the more you do it, the more your experience of the pose shifts to freedom. It is great practice to rotate your shoulders away from your ears while bearing weight in your upper body. As your body awareness grows, you will experience length, strength, and softening all at once. In a flow sequence, it's a time to return to your ujjayi breath, to open your spine and hamstrings, and to open and strengthen tight ankles.

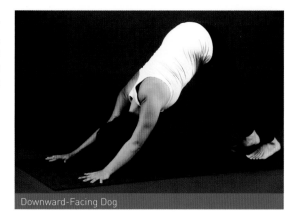
Downward-Facing Dog

SETUP On your hands and knees, point your index finger to the front edge of your mat, or midnight on a clock. Tuck your toes and lift your hips to the sky. • Move your feet back about six inches toward the back edge of your mat. Your hands and feet should be about the same distance from each other as Plank.

ALIGNMENT Point your index fingers to the front of your mat. • Flatten your palms until the knuckles at the base of your index and middle fingers are grounded on your mat. • Move your feet to hip-width distance. Spin your inner ankles back so the outer edges of your feet are parallel with the edge of your mat. • Bend your knees and lift your tailbone toward the ceiling until your spine lengthens. • Spin your sit bones to the wall behind you. • Roll your shoulders up to your ears, then use your back muscles to pull your shoulders down your back and in toward your spine. Squeeze your upper arms toward each other. • Press your chest toward your thighs; keep your shoulders engaged and do not hyperextend in your shoulders if you are extra flexible. • Drive your heels toward the floor (they don't need to touch the floor). • Pull your belly in toward your spine. • Lift the muscles just above your knees to engage your thighs and open into your hamstrings. • Create a long line from your wrists to your shoulders and hips; bend your knees as you need to.

GAZE & FOCUS Look backward at the floor between your big toes. • Lift your tailbone high toward the ceiling.

DEEPEN Once the pose feels more comfortable, press your heels deeply toward the mat until your toes can spread and soften.

COMMON CHALLENGES Tight hamstrings can lead to a rounded spine. • If you have a wrist injury, it may be painful to stay on your hands.

MODIFICATIONS For tight hamstrings, bend your knees and lift your tailbone toward the ceiling. Pull your shoulders toward your spine. Press your chest toward your legs without hyperextending in your shoulders. • For wrist pain, come down to your elbows for Dolphin pose: Bend your elbows so they are stacked directly under your shoulders. Walk your feet in toward your elbows as close as you can. Lift your tailbone to the ceiling.

SEQUENCE TRANSITION From Downward-Facing Dog, walk your feet to your hands.

Rag Doll

Rag Doll releases compression in your spine through gravity. The pose also connects you to your feet and legs, grounding into the lower half of your body and releasing your hamstrings, all areas that can use release after a climb.

SETUP Place your feet hip-width distance apart. Stretch out your toes and activate your feet. Fold your chest toward the floor. Hold your elbows and hang your upper body, letting your head go.

ALIGNMENT Lift and spread out your toes, creating gaps between every toe from your big toe to your pinky toe. • Soften your toes to the floor. Press the four corners of your feet—your big toe and pinky toe knuckles, and the two sides of your heels—into the floor. • Spin your inner ankles toward the back of your mat and energetically draw your outer ankles toward the floor. • Bend your knees slightly until your belly comes down to the tops of your thighs. Squeeze your inner thighs up toward your pelvis. • Turn your head side to side to soften your neck.

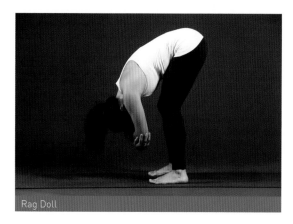

Rag Doll

Stick out your tongue to release your jaw. • Sway gently side to side.

GAZE & FOCUS Close your eyes or set your gaze on a spot between your feet. • Release your spine and neck.

DEEPEN As you get more open in your hamstrings and lower back, your legs straighten more. Keep your knee joints soft still in the pose.

Halfway Lift

A transition pose, Halfway Lift builds strength in your lower back when you hold the pose. It also teaches you to activate your core while hinging at your hips, the biggest joint in your body. In turn, you activate your hamstrings and glutes.

SETUP From Rag Doll, release your hands to the floor. Bring your big toes together. Place your hands on your shins. Lift your chest parallel to the floor.

ALIGNMENT Root your feet firmly into the floor. Bend your knees as needed and squeeze your thighs. • Stick your butt out toward the wall behind you. Lift your chest even with your hips. • Lengthen the crown of your head away from your tailbone. • Hug your shoulder blades together to spine to activate your centerline. Pull your belly up and in.

RELEASE Fold forward to your feet and exhale.

GAZE & FOCUS Look at a spot on the floor in front of your toes. • Create extension in your spine and wrap

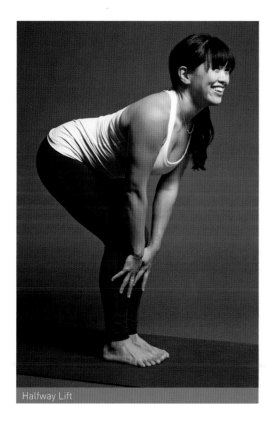
Halfway Lift

your shoulder blades toward your spine. Engage your core.

DEEPEN Place your fingers or hands flat on the floor on the outsides of your feet.

COMMON CHALLENGES Your back rounds because of tight hamstrings.

MODIFICATION Bend your knees. Place your hands above your knees on your thighs or on a block in front of your feet.

Mountain Pose

If you were to set your sights on mastering any pose, make it Mountain Pose. This aptly titled pose holds the key to the universe of yoga poses, teaching neutral alignment of the feet, legs, pelvis, core, shoulders, and spine. Like its namesake, it starts with a broad, strong foundation and rises through your core to lengthen through the top of your head. Once you have mastered the pose, it will bring extraordinary power to your practice and your climbing.

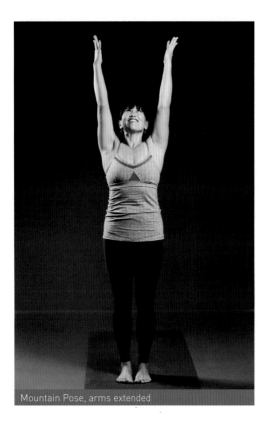
Mountain Pose, arms extended

SETUP Come to standing, with your feet directly underneath your hips, outer edges of your feet parallel to your mat, arms relaxed by your sides.

ALIGNMENT Point your toes straight ahead, and bring the outer edges of your feet parallel with the edges of your mat; you may observe a slight pigeon-toe. Lift your toes and connect with the four corners of your feet to the mat. Soften your toes back to the floor. • Lift the arches of your feet, and with your feet grounded, press your outer shins out until you feel your legs engage and with your feet grounded, spiral your inner ankles toward the back of your mat. Energetically, drive your outer ankles down to the floor. • Squeeze your thigh muscles to the bone. If your knees became stiff, soften the joints slightly. • Tilt your tailbone down toward the floor. Gently pull in your belly button to engage your core. Squeeze your front ribs toward each other. • Roll your shoulders up to your ears, then soften them down away from your ears. Pull your upper arm bones toward your shoulder blades to engage your shoulders. • Contract the muscles under your shoulder blades. Send breath into your ribs in your mid-back. • Let your hands relax by your sides, and spin your palms to face forward. • Extended arms: Reach your arms up to the ceiling in line with your shoulders. Spin your palms to face inward with your thumbs toward the back of your mat. Stretch your fingers out wide. • Lift the crown of your head up toward the sky to lengthen your neck. Soften your jaw. • Set your gaze on one point. • Take ten deep ujjayi breaths.

GAZE & FOCUS Set your eyes at one point in front of you. • Ground your feet and legs, relax your shoulders, and breathe deeply.

VINYASA: BREATH AND MOVEMENT

A flow practice builds heat by connecting breath and poses in your practice. Challenge yourself to breathe according to the sequence of Sun Salutation A and B. As your body tunes in to the practice, notice what shifts in your experience of the flow.

Sun Salutation A

At this point in Strength Practice I, you have already learned all the poses for a Sun Salutation A. This sequence links poses together with cues and breaths for each pose. It builds heat in your body and is a powerful way to warm up your spine and to focus on your breath and the foundational elements of the practice. Repeat the entire sequence three times.

Mountain Pose, inhale with arms up. • Forward Fold, exhale. • Halfway Lift, inhale. • Plank lowered to floor, exhale. • Low Cobra, inhale. • Downward-Facing Dog, exhale, hold pose for five breaths.
• Step or jump forward. • Halfway Lift, inhale.
• Forward Fold, exhale. • Mountain Pose, inhale.

Sun Salutation B

Your body has now warmed up with Sun Salutation A. The Sun Salutation B sequence goes deeper into your leg strength and builds even more internal fire for the next series of standing poses with two new poses: **Chair** and **Warrior I**, described below. Do three full rounds of Sun Salutation B as follows.

Chair, inhale with arms up. (First round: hold for five breaths.) • Forward Fold, exhale. • Halfway Lift, inhale. • Plank to floor, exhale. • Low Cobra, inhale. • Downward-Facing Dog, exhale. • Warrior 1, right side, inhale. (First round: hold for five breaths.) • Plank to floor, exhale. • Low Cobra, inhale • Downward-Facing Dog, exhale. • Warrior 1, left side, inhale. (First round: hold for five breaths.) • Plank to floor, exhale. • Low Cobra, inhale. • Downward-Facing Dog, exhale. Hold pose for five breaths. • Step or jump forward to the front of your mat. • Halfway Lift, inhale. • Forward Fold, exhale.

NEW POSES FOR SUN SALUTATION B

Chair

Contrary to its name, Chair is hardly restful. Without a chair underneath you, you build strength in your legs and your core, with particular strength in hamstrings, quads, glutes, core, and your shoulder girdle. Gravity is your main

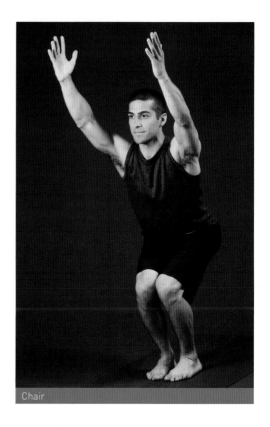

Chair

source of resistance, and this pose builds heat! Remember to breathe.

SETUP Stand with your feet together on your mat (ankles and heels may be slightly apart). Lower your hips toward the floor until you feel your legs engage. Reach your arms up to the ceiling, parallel to your ears with palms facing toward each other. • Activate your core lock and lift your chest toward the ceiling.

ALIGNMENT Keep your toes soft and in view just past your knees. • Spread out your toes. Lift the arches of your feet off the mat and spin your inner ankles toward the back of your mat. • Squeeze your inner thighs toward each other. • Tilt your tailbone toward the floor. Pull your belly in to activate your core. • Lift your chest over your hips and pull your front ribs together. • Soften your shoulders down away from your ears. Engage your back to pull your shoulder blades toward the centerline. • Straighten your arms, stretch out your palms and spread your fingers wide toward the ceiling.

GAZE & FOCUS Lift your eyes off the floor and look at a spot on the wall in front of you. • Focus on strength in your legs and a strong lift in your chest toward the ceiling.

DEEPEN Sink your hips deeper toward the floor. Keep your spine lifted toward the ceiling.

COMMON CHALLENGES Weak quadriceps may pull your knees away from each other. • Tight shoulders prevent you from bringing your arms directly overhead.

MODIFICATIONS Lift the arches of your feet to hug your knees toward each other. • Bend your elbows even with your shoulders at 90-degree angles like a cactus. Hug your shoulder blades together to engage your shoulders. Squeeze your front ribs in toward each other.

Warrior 1

Warrior poses are intentionally challenging. Warrior 1 is the first you will encounter—it is a foundational pose in Sun Salutation B. The pose opens and strengthens your ankles and your hip flexors. It also builds your hamstring strength.

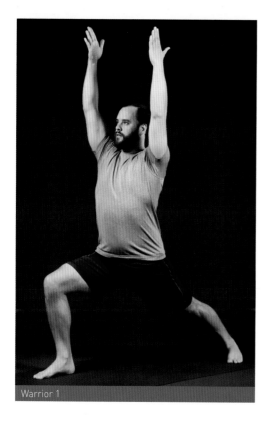
Warrior 1

In addition, your core engagement and shoulder awareness will grow. It is a whole body posture that will challenge you in a new way. While the fundamentals may get easier as you get stronger, you can constantly adjust and refine alignment to challenge yourself.

SETUP From Downward-Facing Dog, step your right foot next to your right thumb. Spin your left heel down and ground it into the mat. Lift your arms up to the ceiling.

ALIGNMENT Point your back foot out about 60 degrees on your mat, with your toes slightly in front of your back heel. • Press the outer edge of your back foot into the mat to connect all four corners of your foot to the floor. • Align your feet so your heels are in one line. Point your front foot toward the front of your mat. Bend your front knee over your ankle. • Spin the hip of your back leg toward the front of your mat while still grounding your back foot. You will feel an opening in your back hip flexor. • Lift your belly button in toward your spine. Squeeze your front ribs toward each other. • Soften your shoulders away from your ears, and squeeze your shoulder blades toward your spine. Reach your arms to the ceiling, keeping your arm bones parallel with your ears. • Stretch out your hands toward the ceiling; spread out your fingers.

GAZE & FOCUS Set your gaze on a wall in front of you. • Squeeze your back leg straight. Hug your core in and up toward your centerline.

DEEPEN Lengthen your stance and bend your front knee to a 90-degree angle.

COMMON CHALLENGES Tight hip flexors and psoas prevent you from bending your front knee to 90 degrees and pull at your lower back. • Tight ankles prevent you from grounding your back foot. • Knee injury prevents you from keeping your heel grounded on your back foot.

MODIFICATIONS Shorten your stance slightly for both challenges until your ankle and hip flexors become more mobile. • If you have a knee injury, lift your back heel for Crescent Lunge (see Strength Practice II).

HEALTHY, HAPPY KNEES

A common misalignment in Warrior 2 and Side Angle is to collapse in your front knee. Weak or tight hips and butt muscles can cause your front knee to collapse inward. The collapse puts unhealthy pressure on your knee joint, an area that already needs all the support it can get to stay strong and stable balance while you are on the wall.

In Warrior 2, squeeze your thigh bones toward your centerline and stack your front knee over your ankle. In Side Angle, the action intensifies. Pull your front thigh bone into your hip socket and squeeze your front outer hip and butt cheek to keep your knee stacked. The alignment will build strength in your glutes, inner thighs, and thigh muscles, and your poses will become strong and grounded.

SEQUENCE TRANSITION Complete Sun Salutation B through the final Forward Fold at the front of your mat.

STRENGTH

The next series of standing poses build strength and power throughout your body. Twists open your spine and chest, while holding standing poses works the smaller muscles in your joints to create stability.

Gorilla

A big wrist and hand release, Gorilla is a counter pose to Downward-Facing Dog and Plank, and stretches your hands out from the climber hand clench. It releases the impact of weight bearing in your wrists, and in this modern day of constant typing and texting, it's a great release for cramped hands.

SETUP In a Forward Fold, move your feet to hip-width distance. Keep your feet stacked under your hips. Slide the palms of your hands underneath your feet—the top of your hands are touching your mat.

ALIGNMENT Wiggle your hands deeper under your feet until your toes reach your wrists. • Bend your elbows to the outer edges of your mat. • Hug your

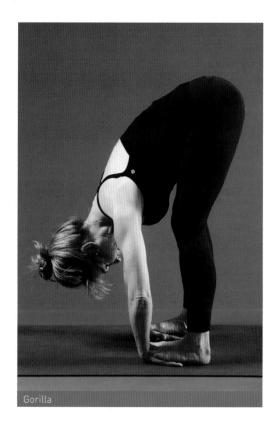

Gorilla

shoulder blades together. Pull your chest deeper toward your spine. • Soften your knees and bring your belly down to your thighs. Engage your thigh muscles. • Release your neck and hang your head toward the floor.

GAZE & FOCUS Look at the floor behind your feet. • Engage your shoulders and back muscles to pull your chest closer to your shins.

DEEPEN Work your legs as straight as your hamstrings allow while still squeezing your thighs. Keep your knee joints soft.

COMMON CHALLENGES Tight hamstrings prevent you from sliding your hands under your feet.

MODIFICATION Make fists and place the tops of your hands on a block, curled fingers facing in toward your body. Bend your knees.

SEQUENCE TRANSITION Release your hands from under your feet. • Bring your feet together. • Stand in Mountain Pose.

Twisted Chair

A powerful twist to release your spine, this twisting add-on to the already energetic Chair gives you a major strength boost in your legs! Twisting poses also teach you to rotate your spine through your mid-back, and will translate to twisting more effectively for complex moves on the wall. Hang on through this one.

SETUP Bring your toes together and lower your hips into Chair. Connect your palms together in front of your chest. On your exhale, twist to the right, hooking your left elbow outside your right knee.

ALIGNMENT Soften your toes and ground the four corners of your feet into the floor. • Make sure your knees stay even; knees askew are an indicator you are popping out a hip to one side. • Lift your right elbow up to the ceiling; press through your hands to deepen your twist. • Pull your belly in toward your spine and stick your sit bones out behind you. • Stretch your chest and head forward, pulling your shoulder blades toward your spine.

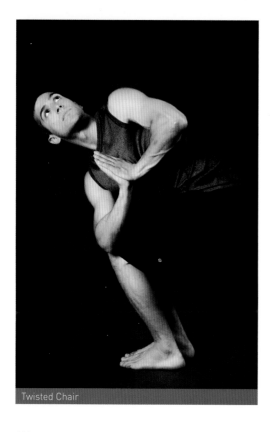

Twisted Chair

GAZE & FOCUS Look up at the ceiling past your upper hand. • Keep your knees even and aligned throughout the twist.

DEEPEN Open your lower hand to a block just outside your right foot. Extend your upper hand to the ceiling, palm facing the same direction as your chest. • Settle your hips lower toward the floor. Hug your inner thighs toward each other and rotate your upper ribs to the ceiling.

COMMON CHALLENGES A lack of torso rotation prevents you from reaching your lower hand outside your foot.

MODIFICATION Bring the block just in front of your feet to support the extension in your twist.

SEQUENCE TRANSITION Release your chest forward to your feet. • Inhale and lengthen your chest to Halfway Lift.

Low Lunge

A modified Crescent Lunge, Low Lunge minimizes the factors of balance and strength. Our hip flexors shorten from sitting all day, and are in constant use when walking. Use this lunge to give your hip flexors some space.

SETUP From Halfway Lift, step your left foot to the back edge of your mat. Lower your back knee to the floor. Point your back toes. Bring your hands to your front thigh.

ALIGNMENT Square your hips toward the front of your mat. Pull your front foot and back knee toward each other to integrate. Your hips will lift slightly higher than before. • Once your centerline is established, slowly shift your weight forward toward your front foot. Stack your front knee over your ankle. • Squeeze your belly in toward your spine and hug your front ribs together. • Reach your arms up toward the ceiling, palms facing in. Breathe deeply into the stretch in your hip flexor.

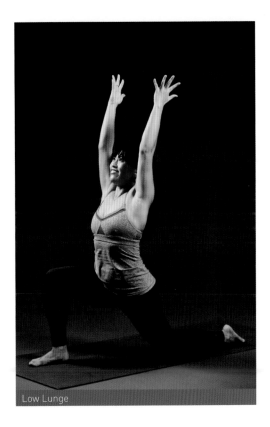

Low Lunge

GAZE & FOCUS Look at a spot on the wall in front of you. • Hug your inner thighs toward each other to keep your body strong while opening into your hip.

DEEPEN Tuck your back toes for a full Crescent Lunge. Lift your back knee off the floor. Squeeze your inner thighs toward your pelvis. Lift your back leg straight.

COMMON CHALLENGES Your knee hurts from being on the ground.

MODIFICATION Fold over an edge of your mat to pad your knee.

Twisted Crescent Lunge

A deep twist that challenges balance, Twisted Crescent Lunge opens your hip flexors, builds strength in your legs, and supports an opening twist in your spine. The pose builds stability in your lower body and releases your spine, important tools for keeping your balance while rotating on the wall.

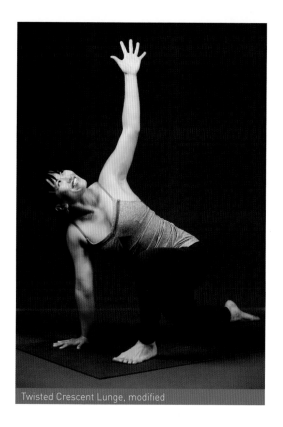

Twisted Crescent Lunge, modified

SETUP From Low Lunge, bring your palms together in front of your chest. Lengthen your chest on an inhale. Exhale and hook your right elbow over your left knee. If you need a block, set it inside your front foot.

ALIGNMENT Shift your weight forward toward your left foot, keeping your knee pointing forward over your ankle; don't let it cave in or out. • Lift your left elbow toward the sky; press down into your palms. • Lengthen your spine through the crown of your head to create more space for the twist. • Hug your shoulder blades toward your spine, and deepen your twist. • Pull your belly in toward your spine. • Bring your lower hand to the floor, or a block inside your front leg. Stretch your upper fingers out wide and toward the ceiling.

GAZE & FOCUS Set your gaze on a spot on the ceiling. • Squeeze your shoulder blades toward each other. Engage the muscles underneath your shoulder blades to deepen your twist.

DEEPEN Tuck your back toes to the ball of your foot and lift your back leg off the floor. Bring your lower hand to the floor or a block outside your front leg.

COMMON CHALLENGES You will need to develop strength and stability in your legs to hold the full pose. Squeeze your inner thighs for balance.

MODIFICATION Keep your back knee on the floor. Pad your knee if you feel pain in your kneecap.

SEQUENCE TRANSITION Bring both hands to the floor on either side of your front foot in a Low Lunge. • Tuck your back toes and spin your back heel down to the floor. • Stack your chest over your hips for Warrior 2.

Warrior 2

Warrior poses rely on your leg strength, and are a good place to explore the balance of effort and ease. Warrior 2 offers great strength, building your quads and hamstrings to keep you strong on the wall. It also teaches you to set your gaze, soften your shoulders, and breathe deeply into the challenge.

SETUP Point your right foot toward the front edge of your mat. Open your toes on your back foot to a 90-degree angle, but no wider than that, from your front foot. Turn your chest to face the same direction as your hips. Reach your arms toward the front and back of your mat parallel to the floor.

ALIGNMENT Stack your front knee over your ankle. (Widen your feet if your knee is bending past the top of your ankle.) • Lift the inner arch of your back foot off the floor. • Pull your feet toward each other to activate your inner thighs toward your pelvis. • Press your front heel firmly into the mat. • Stack your chest over your hips. Lengthen your tailbone down toward the floor. Lift your belly button in toward your spine. • Release your shoulders away from your ears. Pull your arm bones in toward your centerline. Hover your arms parallel to the floor. • From your spine, stretch your fingers to the front and back walls.

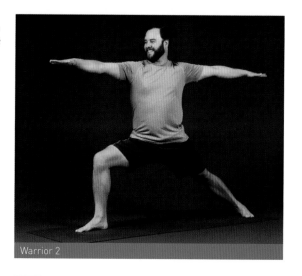

Warrior 2

GAZE & FOCUS Turn your head toward your front hand and set your gaze at your fingertips. • Squeeze your thigh bones in toward each other. Relax your jaw and eyes.

DEEPEN Widen your stance and bend your right knee to a 90-degree angle over your front ankle.

COMMON CHALLENGES Weak or tight outer hips and glutes can cause your front knee to collapse inward rather than staying stacked over your front ankle.

MODIFICATIONS Shorten your stance. Keep your knee aligned over your front ankle to build strength and prevent injury.

SEQUENCE TRANSITION From Warrior 2, straighten your front leg.

Triangle

A powerful grounding pose, Triangle relies on the bones of your body to open and strengthen. You'll get into your deeper psoas muscle in your hip; lengthen your hamstrings; and create a long, neutral spine. Triangle pose gives you greater stability against gravity and encourages a deeper listening to your body. Challenge yourself by moving your drishti to the ceiling.

SETUP With both legs straight, extend your front hand toward the front of your mat until your torso is parallel to the floor. Shift your front hip toward the back of your mat. Place your right hand on your front shin or on a block outside your right foot. Reach your upper hand toward the ceiling.

ALIGNMENT Ground the four corners of both feet into the floor. • Pull your front thigh bone up into your hip socket; your back hip will roll slightly forward toward the floor. • Lift the top of your right kneecap to lengthen into your hamstrings. Keep a slight bend in your front knee so you don't lock or hyperextend into the joint. • Hug your shoulders in toward your spine. • Stretch your chest toward the front of your mat; spin your upper ribs toward the ceiling. Stretch out your fingers on your upper hand.

GAZE & FOCUS Look up at the ceiling and set your gaze on one spot. • Press your big toe knuckle of your front foot into the floor. Focus on the stability of your legs and length in your spine.

DEEPEN Widen your stance. Reach your lower hand deeper toward your ankle or the floor.

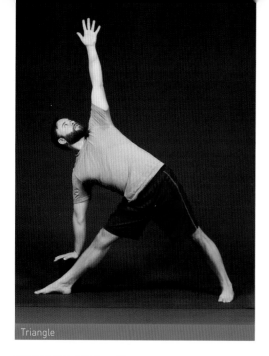

Triangle

MODIFICATION Use a block at the tallest height outside your front foot. If necessary, stack two blocks to get enough height to lengthen your spine. • Soften your front knee joint and lift the muscles above your knee.

SEQUENCE TRANSITION From Triangle, come up to Warrior 2. • Bend your front leg for Side Angle.

Side Angle

If I were permitted to have a favorite pose, it would be this one. One of the most challenging standing poses when done with proper alignment, Side Angle strengthens your glutes and legs and opens your spine. It will test your limits. Take on the challenge.

SETUP Lower your front forearm onto your front thigh. Reach your upper arm up to the ceiling, your palm facing the same direction as your chest.

ALIGNMENT Ground the four corners of both feet into the floor. Squeeze both feet toward the center

COMMON CHALLENGES Tight hamstrings or a tight psoas prevent you from reaching your shin. • You overextend in your front knee joint.

of your mat. • Stack your front knee over your front ankle. • Pull your front thigh bone into your hip socket until you feel your outer glute engage.
• Keep your right hip even with your bent front knee.
• Lift the arch of your back foot and squeeze your back inner thigh. • Engage your belly to lighten the weight of your front arm on your thigh. • Pull your shoulder blades toward your spine. Spiral your upper ribs up toward the ceiling. • Spread out your fingers on both hands.

GAZE & FOCUS Set your gaze on your upper finger-tips. • Squeeze your front hip and bend your front leg deeper.

DEEPEN Lower your front hand to a block or the floor just inside your front foot. Extend your upper arm in a diagonal line forward.

COMMON CHALLENGES Weak glutes cause your front knee to collapse inward.

MODIFICATION Shorten your stance slightly as long as you keep your front knee aligned over your ankle.

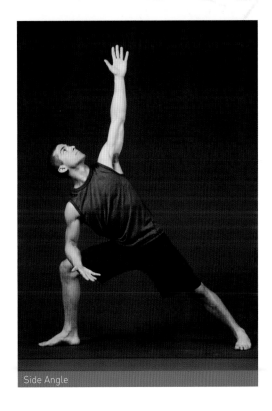
Side Angle

SEQUENCE TRANSITION Connect through a Vinyasa: Bring both hands to the floor for Plank. • Shift forward and lower to the floor on an exhale. • Lift your chest for Low Cobra, inhale. • Tuck your toes and lift your hips to the sky for Downward-Facing Dog on an exhale. • Step or jump to the front of your mat. • Repeat the poses on the left side from Twisted Chair to Side Angle. • Step to the front of your mat for Balancing Poses.

BALANCING

Climbers must master balance to climb well. Unlike the wall where tiny toe-holds require nimble feet, focus on grounding into all four corners of your standing foot in your yoga poses. You will stabilize your feet, ankles, and knees and keep them healthy for challenging climbing moves.

Eagle

A balancing pose that generates from your centerline, Eagle builds balance and requires concentration and focus. Squeeze your inner thighs for strength and observe how the arm bind opens shoulders tight from climbing.

SETUP Stand in Mountain Pose, extend your arms out wide and parallel to the floor, palms facing forward. Cross your right upper arm underneath your left upper arm. Wind your forearms around each other. Bring your palms to touch for the full bind. Lower into Chair in your legs. Cross your right thigh on top of your left thigh.

ALIGNMENT Ground into your standing foot. Squeeze your inner thighs all the way together. • Stretch out your toes on your upper foot. • Stack your shoulders over your hips; engage your core lock. • Lift your elbows level with your shoulders. Press your hands away from your face to stack your wrists over your elbows. • Soften your shoulders away from your ears; pull your arm bones in toward your shoulder sockets.

GAZE & FOCUS Look past your arms to set your drishti on a spot on the wall. • Engage your belly firmly and set your gaze.

DEEPEN Bend your standing leg deeper and wrap your right foot around your calf. Challenge your balance by moving your gaze in toward your forearms.

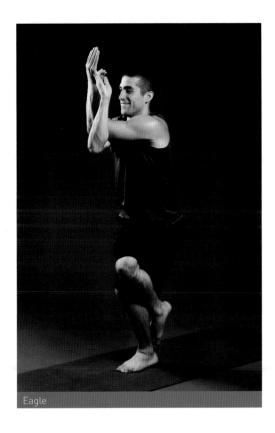
Eagle

COMMON CHALLENGES Tight shoulders can prevent you from taking a full bind.

MODIFICATION Reach for opposite shoulders and lift your elbows even with your shoulders.

SEQUENCE TRANSITION Release into Mountain Pose.
• Do Eagle on the left side; wrap your left arm under your right, and lift your left leg over your right leg.

Tree

Tree pose embodies the art of balancing. Your standing foot spreads wide and stretches into the earth. Your standing leg is straight and strong. When you hug into your core, you can extend your arms and energy up and out. Let go of the worry that you might step out of the pose. Instead, lift your gaze skyward and see what is possible.

SETUP Stand with your feet together in Mountain Pose. Lift your right foot to either your inner calf or above your knee joint to your inner thigh. Bring your palms together at the center of your chest.

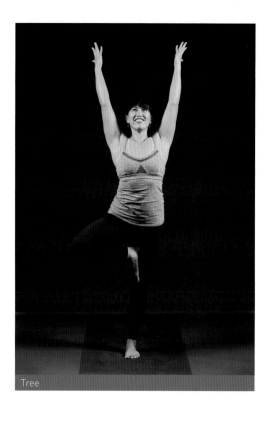
Tree

ALIGNMENT Ground the four corners of your standing foot into your mat. • Press your lifted foot into your standing leg. • Hug your shoulder blades to your spine. Press your palms together. • Pull your belly in toward your spine; lift your lower ribs away from your pelvis. • Lift your hands on an inhale toward the ceiling, palms facing each other.

GAZE & FOCUS Set your gaze on a spot in front of you. Once you are stable, move your drishti up the wall to the ceiling or your hands. • Ground your standing leg and stretch your spine skyward.

DEEPEN Walk your gaze up to a spot on the ceiling behind you.

COMMON CHALLENGES You are still building strength in your feet and have trouble staying upright with only one foot on the floor.

MODIFICATION Prop the foot of your bent leg against the ankle of your standing foot with the ball of your foot on the floor.

Release to Mountain Pose.
• Do Tree on the left side. • From Mountain Pose, reach your arms overhead, inhale. • Fold your chest to your thighs, exhale. • Lift your chest to Halfway Lift, inhale. • Plant your hands and step your feet to Plank. • Roll to the tops of your toes and lower to the floor, exhale. • Lift your chest for Low Cobra, inhale. • Exhale and press back to Downward-Facing Dog.

BACKBENDS

Backbends train your body away from habits including the tendency to roll your chest forward, whether it's sitting during the day or while climbing. By opening your chest, you will shift how you use your shoulders, strengthen your spine, and energize your body.

Flip Dog

A fun backbend, Flip Dog opens your chest and strengthens your shoulder girdle, working the opposite direction of how you use your shoulders while climbing. It looks intimidating, but is surprisingly easy. Let your neck relax once you're there and press into your legs for full strength in the pose.

SETUP From Downward-Facing Dog, lift your right leg to the ceiling. Bend your right knee and roll your hip open for Three-Legged Dog. Look under your left arm for your upper foot and lower it to the floor behind you. Turn your other foot around 180 degrees until both toes are flat and parallel on the ground.
• Keep your left hand where it started on the ground and reach your free arm overhead toward the floor.

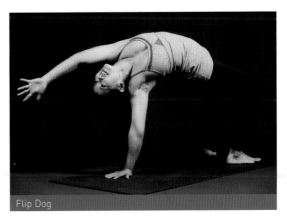

Flip Dog

ALIGNMENT Set your feet hip-width distance.
• Press into the four corners of your feet and lift your hips to the ceiling. • Bend your right elbow even with your shoulder for a cactus arm. Hug your shoulder blades toward each other to open your chest. • Engage your core lock. • Soften your neck to let your head hang toward the floor.

GAZE & FOCUS Set your gaze on the front wall or the floor under you. • Press down into your feet to lift your hips higher. Hug your shoulder blades in toward your spine.

DEEPEN Reach your hand overhead toward the floor.

COMMON CHALLENGES If you have shoulder pain, be mindful in this pose—and skip if it exacerbates the injury.

MODIFICATION Stay in Three-Legged Dog.

SEQUENCE TRANSITION To release, lift your right arm to the ceiling. • Hop back over to Three-Legged Dog. • Lower your upper foot and move forward to Plank. • Bring your feet together, shift your weight into your right hand, and roll to the outer edge of your right foot.

Side Plank

Side Plank brings the art of a static hold to one side of your body. It works the lower side of your body closest to the floor, from your legs to your obliques to your back muscles and shoulders. A strong Side Plank will develop your body's endurance and overall strength for long days climbing.

SETUP Stack your left foot on top of your right foot. Move your right shoulder over your right wrist. Lift your left hand up to the ceiling, palm facing the same direction as your chest.

ALIGNMENT Your right fingers face the front of the mat and your right hand is stacked a couple of inches forward of your shoulder. • Flex your toes toward your knees and squeeze the muscles of your legs to the bone. • Keep your body at one angled plane from shoulders to feet. • Pull your shoulder blades in toward your spine to take the weight out of your wrist. • Spread out the fingers on your upper

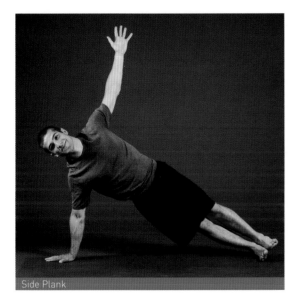
Side Plank

DEEPEN Lift your upper leg as high as you can toward the ceiling.

COMMON CHALLENGES You are still building strength and struggle to hold the pose.

MODIFICATION Bring your lower knee to the floor underneath your hip for support, keeping your foundation of hand, lower knee and feet in one line.

SEQUENCE TRANSITION From Side Plank, bring your upper hand to the floor for Plank. • Shift forward and lower to the floor on an exhale. • Lift to Low Cobra, inhale. • Move to Downward-Facing Dog, exhale. • Do Flip Dog through Side Plank on your left side. • Move forward to Plank. • Exhale and lower to the floor for Bow.

Bow

Strong legs are instrumental to backbends, and Bow pose teaches your body how to engage your legs for backbends, in addition to opening up your quadriceps and strengthening your back.

hand. • Lengthen the crown of your head toward the front of your mat.

GAZE & FOCUS Look at the ceiling. • Create stability through your legs and core.

SETUP From your belly on the floor, bend both knees. Reach for the outer edges of your feet with your hands.

ALIGNMENT Bring your knees to hip-width distance to support your lower back and tap into your leg strength. • Stretch out your toes, and spin your inner ankles toward your lower back. • Pull your belly in toward your spine. • Press your pelvis down toward the floor. Lift your feet up toward the ceiling. • Use your leg strength to lift as high as you can.

GAZE & FOCUS Lift your eyes to the floor or the front of the room. • Engage your core and use your legs in the pose.

DEEPEN Reach for your ankles. Flex your toes and rock back to the tops of your thighs.

COMMON CHALLENGES Tight hamstrings or knee injuries prevent you from grabbing both of your feet at the same time.

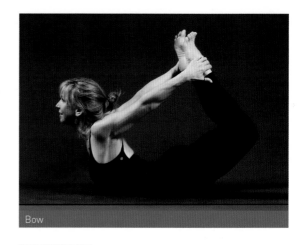
Bow

MODIFICATION Bring your left forearm parallel to the front edge of your mat. Stack your left elbow under your left shoulder, palm facing down on the floor. Reach your right hand to your right foot. Press into your left elbow and lift your right foot up to the ceiling. Do both sides. • Alternative: Substitute with the Locust pose (see Strength Practice II later in this chapter).

Let go of your feet gently. Roll your hips side to side on the floor. • Do a second Bow. • Plant your hands next to your ribs. • Lift to Low Cobra, inhale. • Tuck your toes and come back to Downward-Facing Dog, exhale. • Walk your feet forward between your hands. • Sit down and lower down to your back for Bridge.

Bridge

Despite the temptation to rest on your back, it's not time yet! Bridge is a modification for Wheel, which you will learn in Strength Practice II. More importantly, this backbend teaches you to use your legs and to open your chest by integrating and opening your spine and shoulders.

SETUP Walk your feet closer to your body until your fingertips brush your heels. Set your feet parallel and hip-width distance. Press into the four corners of your feet to lift your hips to the ceiling. Move your shoulders together and interlace your hands underneath your body.

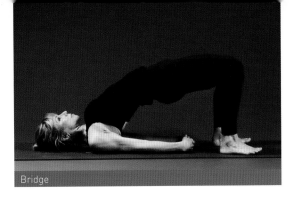

Bridge

ALIGNMENT Press your feet into your mat until your legs engage. • Stack your knees over your ankles. • Spin your inner thighs toward each other and down toward your mat. • Position your hands at your spine just above the tailbone. Feel the ridge of muscles around your spine engage. Lift until you feel your spine engage between your shoulder blades. Press your interlaced hands into the floor. • Pull your chest toward the back wall. • Squeeze your front ribs together.

RELEASE Reach your arms up to the ceiling. Slowly release your spine toward the floor, one vertebrae at a time.

GAZE & FOCUS Look at a spot on the ceiling. • Press deeply into your feet for strong legs.

DEEPEN Lift your right knee into your chest. Press strongly into your rooted foot. Extend your right leg, foot flexed, to the ceiling, keeping your hips level. Switch sides.

COMMON CHALLENGES Tight shoulders prevent you from interlacing your hands.

MODIFICATION Use a strap between your hands for a bind. Or press your palms into the floor.

SEQUENCE TRANSITION Reach your arms to the ceiling to slowly release down. • Do a second Bridge. • Lower your hips to the floor for Reclined Half Pigeon.

RECOVER AND RESTORE
The end of a practice gives your body time to soften and relax. Throughout these final poses, notice how your body sensations and your mental state have shifted through the practice.

Reclined Half Pigeon

Reclined Half Pigeon is a supported way to open your muscular hip region. Hip opening can be an intense experience—there is no need to force the opening, but rather surrender into it. Breathe deeply and move gently to deepen into the pose.

SETUP With your feet flat on the floor, cross your right ankle over your left knee. Keep your right foot flexed toward your knee to protect your knee joint.

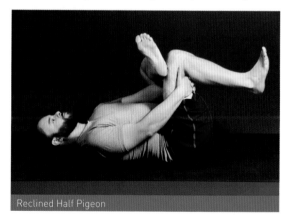

Reclined Half Pigeon

Reach your right hand between your legs and your left hand behind your left thigh to support it, and pull your legs toward your chest.

ALIGNMENT Pull your left leg toward you to get a deep stretch in your outer right hip. • Relax your shoulders toward the floor. • Press your right elbow into your right inner thigh to deepen the stretch. • Take ten deep breaths.

GAZE & FOCUS Close your eyes or look at a spot on the ceiling. • Notice the sensations in your hip and breathe into it to release the muscles.

DEEPEN Straighten your free leg up to the ceiling and press through your heel.

COMMON CHALLENGES Tight hips prevent you from holding the back of your leg.

MODIFICATION Take a strap around the back of your left leg, and pull your leg toward your chest.

SEQUENCE TRANSITION Release your legs from Half Pigeon. • Repeat Reclined Half Pigeon on your left side. • Pull your knees into your chest. • Using momentum, rock yourself up to a seated position.

Seated Forward Fold

Gravity comes into play in all forward folds as you pull your torso toward your legs. In a Seated Forward Fold, you also stretch your calves, hamstrings, glutes, and the muscles along your spine—a stretch that feels exceptionally good after many hours of climbing.

SETUP From your seated position, extend your legs straight to the front of your mat. • Reach your hands toward the outer edges of your feet.

ALIGNMENT Flex your toes toward your knees. • Contract your quad muscles to the bone. • Pull your chest toward your feet and lengthen your lower back. • Relax your head.

FOCUS Lengthen your chest toward your feet. Extend from your lower spine.

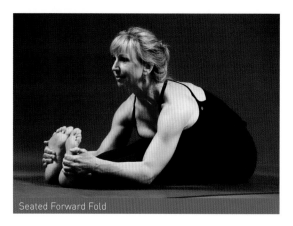
Seated Forward Fold

MODIFICATIONS Place a block or blanket underneath your sit bones to relax your hips and core for the forward fold. Alternatively, bend your knees to reach for your feet, or use a strap to lengthen your reach to your feet to allow your hips flexors and core to relax.

Seated Twist

Final twists, such as this Seated Twist, release the spine after the intensity of a practice. They relax your spine while also working into a natural rotation.

DEEPEN Press the backs of your knees toward the floor without overextending the joint, and squeeze your quads. If your hands reach past your feet, use a block at the soles of your feet to give you more room to deepen.

COMMON CHALLENGES A tight lower back, hamstrings, or hip flexors can tend to contract and prevent your torso from folding forward.

SETUP From Seated Forward Fold, extend your right leg straight to the front of your mat, toes flexed. Place your left foot on the floor outside your right thigh. Place your left hand on the floor behind you. Reach your right arm up to the ceiling. Wrap your right arm around your bent leg.

ALIGNMENT Lengthen your spine on your inhale. Twist toward your bent leg on your exhale.

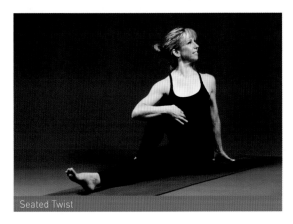
Seated Twist

GAZE & FOCUS Move your gaze past your left shoulder. • Inhale to lengthen your spine and exhale to deepen your twist. Do not force the twist.

DEEPEN Hook your right elbow outside your left leg. Cross your lower leg underneath you.

SEQUENCE TRANSITION To release, come back to center. • Repeat the twist on the right side. • Bring your feet to the floor and lower down to your back.

Legs Up the Wall

Inversions allow gravity to lighten the load your heart usually takes on to pull blood up from your legs. Legs Up the Wall lets gravity do the work and is a restorative pose. Feel free to take the name of this pose literally by moving to a wall—or practice it on your mat.

SETUP Walk your feet in and lift your hips like you are going to Bridge pose. Position a block at its lowest height underneath your sacrum. Set your hips down, adjusting the block to find a comfortable resting point. • Lift your legs to the ceiling.

ALIGNMENT Flex your toes toward your knees. • Relax your shoulders, face, and hands.

GAZE & FOCUS Set your drishti on your feet. • Breathe deeply and relax. Keep your legs still.

DEEPEN Choose a more active inversion with Shoulder Stand (see Strength Practice II).

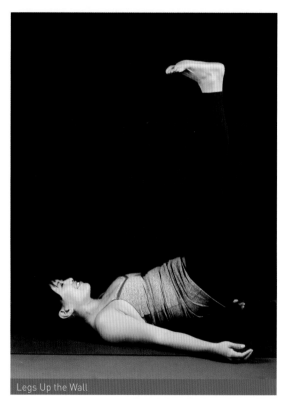

Legs Up the Wall

COMMON CHALLENGES Tight hamstrings make it uncomfortable or difficult to keep your legs vertical.

MODIFICATION Loop a strap over the soles of your feet. Flex your feet. Hold onto the ends of the strap. Bring your elbows to the floor.

SEQUENCE TRANSITION Bring your feet back to the floor. • Lift your hips and move the block aside.

FINAL REST

Some people, especially active folks, can find stillness uncomfortable. Let go of your fidgety side. Take on Final Rest, and be soft and still.

Corpse Pose

Corpse Pose will either be the best pose you have ever tried, or the worst! Commit to closing your eyes and being quiet. If you are cold, cover yourself with a blanket.

SETUP From your back, straighten your legs on your mat. With arms at your sides, turn your palms to face the sky.

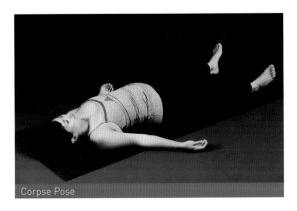

Corpse Pose

ALIGNMENT Slide your shoulders under you.
• Relax the muscles in your legs, shoulders, and face. • Move into your natural breath. • Close your eyes. • Stay in this pose for three minutes.

FOCUS Stay awake and still. Notice your natural breath.

DEEPEN Take a five-minute final rest.

STRENGTH PRACTICE II

TIME: 45 MINUTES
EQUIPMENT: YOGA MAT, BLOCK, AND STRAP

This 45-minute strength sequence builds off the first, adding on more challenge in the early Sun Salutation A and B sequences plus new and added intensity during the standing poses. Once you are comfortable with Strength Practice I, dive in. Or, if you are ready for a challenge, take on this practice now!

All poses should be held for five breaths unless otherwise noted.

RELEASE AND ACTIVATE

Lying on your back sends a signal to your brain to relax. Let go of any tension in your body at the beginning of your practice. Bring in your ujjayi breath before you start.

Supine Butterfly

As you learned in Strength Practice I, Supine Butterfly activates your hips and sends a signal to your brain that all is well.

SEQUENCE FOR STRENGTH PRACTICE II

- » Supine Butterfly
- » Reclined Half Pigeon
- » Happy Baby
- » Boat
- » Plank
- » Downward-Facing Dog
- » Halfway Lift
- » Sun Salutation A
- » Sun Salutation B
- » Hand-to-Big-Toe Forward Fold

- » Gorilla
- » Twisted Chair
- » Crescent Lunge
- » Twisted Crescent Lunge
- » Warrior 2
- » Triangle
- » Half-Bound Side Angle
- » Wide-Legged Forward Fold
- » Skandasana
- » Squat

- » Crow
- » Eagle
- » Hand-to-Knee Balancing Pose
- » Airplane
- » Half Moon
- » Revolved Triangle
- » Flip Dog
- » Side Plank
- » Locust
- » Bow
- » Bridge

- » Wheel
- » Lizard
- » Half Pigeon
- » Double Pigeon
- » Reverse Tabletop
- » Head-to-Knee Seated Forward Fold
- » Shoulder Stand
- » Ear Pressure Pose
- » Fish
- » Supine Twist
- » Corpse Pose

SETUP Lay down with your back on your mat. Bring the soles of your feet together so your legs form a diamond shape.

ALIGNMENT Let your arms relax on the floor, palms facing up. • Notice the connection of your spine to the floor and the natural curve of your lumbar spine at your lower back. • Hug your belly up and in toward your spine to activate your core. • Bring in your ujjayi breath.

GAZE & FOCUS Close your eyes. • Bring your attention to your spine on the floor and an active core.

COMMON CHALLENGES Tight hips or lower back pain prevent you from relaxing your hips.

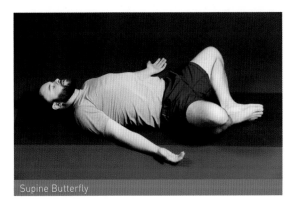

Supine Butterfly

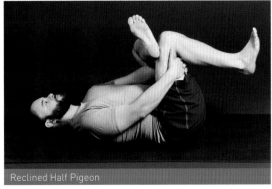

Reclined Half Pigeon

MODIFICATION Bring your feet as wide as your mat and rest your knees together to bring your lower back to the mat.

Reclined Half Pigeon

Create a gentle opening into your hips at the beginning of this practice. Use this time to notice any tension that has built up from sitting or hauling heavy gear for a climb.

SETUP Bring your feet flat to the floor. Cross your right ankle over your left knee. Keep your right foot flexed toward your knee to protect your knee joint.
• Reach your right hand between your legs and your left hand behind your left thigh to support it, and pull your legs toward your chest.

ALIGNMENT Pull your left leg toward you to get a deep stretch in your outer right hip. • Relax your shoulders toward the floor. • Press your right elbow into your right inner thigh to deepen the stretch. • Take ten deep breaths.

GAZE & FOCUS Close your eyes or look at a spot on the ceiling. • Notice the sensations in your hip and breathe into it to release the muscles.

DEEPEN Straighten your free leg up to the ceiling and press through your heel.

COMMON CHALLENGES Tight hips prevent you from holding the back of your leg.

MODIFICATION Take a strap around the back of your left leg, and pull your leg toward your chest.

SEQUENCE TRANSITION Do Reclined Half Pigeon on your left side. • Pull your knees into your chest.

Happy Baby

Open your hips and lengthen your spine and relax. Experiment with the pose by switching your hands between the inner and outer arches of your feet.

SETUP Take your knees wide outside your chest. Reach inside your legs for the inner arches of your feet and lift your feet toward the ceiling.

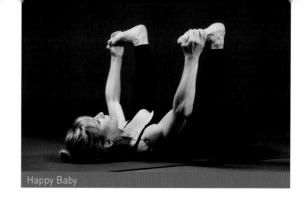
Happy Baby

ALIGNMENT Flex your feet toward your knees. Bend your knees at a 90-degree angle. • Press your heels toward the ceiling. • Relax your shoulders. • Lengthen your lower back toward the floor while pulling on your feet with your hands. • Press your feet into your hands.

GAZE & FOCUS Look at a spot on the ceiling. • Lengthen your spine to the mat.

DEEPEN Switch your grip on your feet to the outside arch of your foot; pull your knees deeper down outside your ribs.

COMMON CHALLENGES Tight hips or lower back prevent you from reaching your feet.

MODIFICATION Hold the backs of your thighs instead of your feet. Open your knees wider than your chest. Place a block under your head.

SEQUENCE TRANSITION From Happy Baby, pull your knees into your chest. • With momentum, rock up to a seated position.

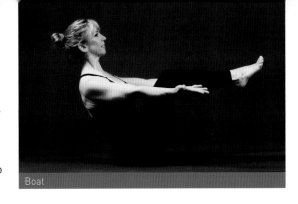

Boat

Boat

Boat accesses deep core muscles that stabilize you even when you don't know it. Challenge yourself in this sequence by taking on additional Low Boats, see variation below.

SETUP From a seated position, hold the backs of your thighs, and balance between your sit bones at the base of your pelvis and your tailbone. Lift your feet off the floor.

ALIGNMENT Pull your thighs toward your chest. Hold your shins parallel to the floor. • Squeeze your thighs toward each other. Spread out your toes so you see a gap between each one. • Pull your shoulder blades toward each other. Lift your chest toward the ceiling. • Reach your arms straight in front of you. • Stay for ten breaths.

LOW BOAT VARIATION Lower your torso and legs until your lower back connects to the floor, your shoulders stay off the floor, and your legs hover off the mat straight ahead. Squeeze your thighs together. Look at your toes. Use your core, and lift back to (High) Boat. • Repeat this cycle five times, holding each variation for five breaths.

GAZE & FOCUS Set your gaze on your toes. • Concentrate on lifting your chest and lengthening your spine.

DEEPEN Once your hamstrings allow it, straighten your legs at a 45-degree angle away from the floor.

COMMON CHALLENGES Lower back weakness prevents you from lifting your chest.

MODIFICATION Hold the back of your thighs to keep your chest lifted.

SEQUENCE TRANSITION Bring your feet to the floor. • Squeeze your knees and lift your chest to release in your abdominal muscles. • Cross your ankles, roll over your feet, and come to your hands and knees for Plank.

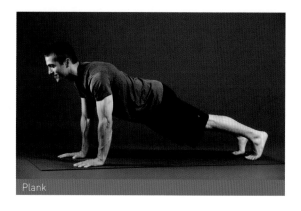

Plank

Plank

Add some heat to your Plank pose with additional variations to fire up your abdominal and back muscles.

SETUP Stack your hands underneath your shoulders, index finger pointed straight ahead. Step your feet to the back of your mat. Stay on the balls of your feet, lift your knees off the floor and squeeze your legs straight.

ALIGNMENT Keep your hips just below level with your shoulders. • Spiral your inner thighs up to the ceiling. Lengthen the backs of your knees and squeeze your thighs. • Lift your head so your neck is level with your shoulders. • Press your palms firmly into the floor. Squeeze your upper arm bones toward each other. • Spin the inner eye of your elbows forward, and pull your shoulder blades together. • Tilt your tailbone toward your heels. • Lift your belly in toward your spine and wrap your front ribs together. • Stay for ten breaths.

PLANK VARIATION I Lift your right foot off the floor three inches, toes flexed. Squeeze your leg muscles, especially in your left leg. Hold for five breaths. Switch legs.

PLANK VARIATION II Bring your right knee to your chest. Keep your hips level with your shoulders and lift your gaze forward. Step your right foot back. • Bring your left knee to your chest. Keep your head lifted. Hug your knee to your chest. • Do both sides three times.

GAZE & FOCUS Set your drishti past the front of your mat. • Keep your legs and core firm. Breathe deeply to maintain the pose.

COMMON CHALLENGES Building strength to hold the full pose for ten breaths can take some practice.

MODIFICATION Bring your knees to the floor, toes curled under. Keep your hips in one even line with your shoulders, core engaged.

SEQUENCE TRANSITION From Plank, lift your hips to the ceiling for Downward-Facing Dog.

Downward-Facing Dog

Strengthen your ankles and open your hips by mixing in a Three-Legged Dog pose with your Downward-Facing Dog. Adding a leg lift and hip rotation also stretches dynamically into your hip, which can always use more attention and space to boost your climbing.

SETUP Keep your hands at shoulder-width distance. Lift your hips up to the ceiling.

ALIGNMENT Point your index fingers to the front of your mat. • Flatten your palms until the knuckles at the base of your index and middle fingers are grounded on your mat. • Move your feet to hip-width distance. Spin your inner ankles back so the outer edges of your feet are parallel with the edge of your mat. • Bend your knees and lift your tailbone toward the ceiling until your spine lengthens. Spin your sit bones to the wall behind you. • Roll your shoulders up to your ears, then use your back muscles to pull your shoulders down your back and in toward your spine. Squeeze your upper arms toward each other. • Press your chest toward your thighs; keep your shoulders engaged and do not hyperextend in your shoulders if you are extra flexible. • Drive your heels toward the floor (they don't need to touch the floor). • Pull your belly in toward your spine. • Lift the muscles just above your knees to engage your thighs and open into your hamstrings. • Create a long line from your wrists to your shoulders and hips; bend your knees as you need to.

GAZE & FOCUS Look backward at the floor between your big toes. • Lift your tailbone high toward the ceiling.

DEEPEN Once the pose feels more comfortable, press your heels deeply toward the mat until your toes can spread and soften.

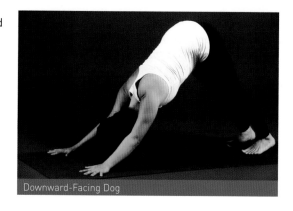
Downward-Facing Dog

COMMON CHALLENGES Tight hamstrings can lead to a rounded spine. • If you have a wrist injury, it may be painful to stay on your hands.

MODIFICATIONS For tight hamstrings, bend your knees and lift your tailbone toward the ceiling. Pull your shoulders toward your spine. Press your chest toward your legs. • For wrist pain, come down to your elbows for Dolphin pose: Bend your elbows so they are stacked directly under your shoulders. Walk your feet in toward your elbows as close as you can. Lift your tailbone to the ceiling.

THREE-LEGGED DOG VARIATION From Downward-Facing Dog, bring your feet together. Lift up your right leg and stretch it toward the wall behind you. Bend your knee and roll your right hip on top of your left. Lift your right knee up to the ceiling.
• Lift your upper knee another three inches toward the ceiling. Keep your shoulders squared to the floor. • Keep your left shoulder level with your right. Stay for five breaths. • **Gaze:** Set your gaze on the back of your mat.

SEQUENCE TRANSITION Do Three-Legged Dog on the right side. • Repeat on the left side. • Lower your upper leg to the floor. Step or hop to the front of your mat. Bring your feet together.

Halfway Lift

An inhale moves you into an extension of your spine in this Halfway Lift pose. Lead with your breath to create more space between your vertebrae and to strengthen your lower back and core. Bend your knees to ensure you are hinging at your hips.

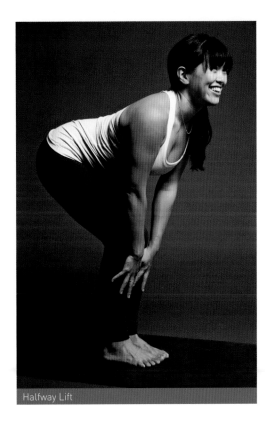
Halfway Lift

SETUP Bring your hands to your shins. Lift your chest parallel to the floor. Squeeze your shoulder blades to your spine. Hug your belly muscles in toward your back, and lift your chest parallel to the floor.

ALIGNMENT Root your feet firmly into the floor. Bend your knees as needed and squeeze your thighs. • Stick your butt out toward the wall behind you. Lift your chest even with your hips. • Lengthen the crown of your head away from your tailbone. • Hug your shoulder blades together to spine to activate your centerline. Pull your belly in and up.

GAZE & FOCUS Look at a spot on the floor in front of your toes. • Create extension in your spine and wrap your shoulder blades toward your spine. Engage your core.

DEEPEN Place your fingers or hands flat on the floor on the outsides of your feet.

COMMON CHALLENGES Your back rounds because of tight hamstrings.

MODIFICATION Bend your knees. Place your hands above your knees on your thighs or on a block in front of your feet.

SEQUENCE TRANSITION Fold forward toward your feet to release.

VINYASA: BREATH AND MOVEMENT

The following flow practice intensifies with the addition of Chaturanga and Upward-Facing Dog in Sun Salutation A and B. Challenge yourself to continue breathing according to the sequences to build strength, heat, and lung capacity.

Sun Salutation A

You will follow roughly the same sequence for Sun Salutation A as you did in Strength Practice I, but add **Chaturanga** and **Upward-Facing Dog**, described below. Do this sequence three times.

Mountain Pose, inhale with arms up. • Forward Fold, exhale. • Halfway Lift, inhale. • Chaturanga, exhale. • Upward-Facing Dog, inhale. • Downward-Facing Dog, exhale, five breaths. • Step or jump to the front of your mat. • Halfway Lift, inhale. • Forward Fold, exhale. • Mountain Pose, inhale.

NEW POSES FOR SUN SALUTATION A

Chaturanga (Low Plank)

A low plank, as Chaturanga is sometimes called, is a step up from the strength needed to lower with control to the floor in Strength Practice I. Chaturanga strengthens your legs, torso, arms, and wrists, and yet many people overrely on shoulder ligaments rather than big trunk muscles for strength. Learn to integrate your shoulders into your spine through Mountain Pose and Plank to balance shoulders strong from climbing, and to develop a powerful Chaturanga.

SETUP From Plank, the fourth pose in Sun Salutation A, roll forward in the pose until you're on the tops of your toes. Lower your body in a strong plank, your core strong and active, until your shoulders are even with your elbows.

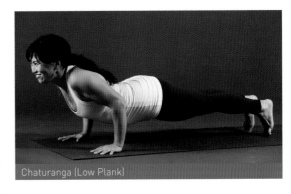
Chaturanga (Low Plank)

ALIGNMENT Squeeze your thigh muscles to the bone. • Pull your shoulder blades toward your spine to keep your chest open. • Engage your core as you lower. • Tilt your tailbone toward your heels to engage your front ribs and core muscles. • Point your elbows to the back of your mat, keeping them about two inches or so away from your ribs and stacked directly over your wrists. • Ensure your shoulders are even with your elbows at a 90-degree angle. If that is difficult to hold, stop with your shoulders slightly higher than your elbows. *Do not dip below 90 degrees.* • Practice lowering from Plank into Chaturanga with a one-breath exhale.

GAZE & FOCUS Look past the front edge of your mat.
• Squeeze your shoulder blades together, and use your back and belly muscles to hold.

DEEPEN Hold Chaturanga for five breaths.

COMMON CHALLENGES Weakness in core and shoulders leads to shoulders rolling forward toward your mat or dropping below a 90-degree angle.

MODIFICATION Bring your knees to the floor. Keep your hips in one diagonal line with your shoulders and lower to a 90-degree bend in your elbows. To modify further, lower to the floor.

Upward-Facing Dog

A backbend that develops strength in your back and shoulders, energizes your spine, and opens your chest, Upward-Facing Dog is strong and fiery.

SETUP From Chaturanga, roll onto the tops of your feet. Pull your chest forward and up to the ceiling and straighten your arms. Stack your shoulders over your wrists.

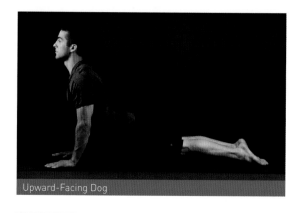
Upward-Facing Dog

ALIGNMENT Press the tops of your toes into your mat. • Lift your knees off the floor and press the pinky toe edge of your feet into the floor; squeeze your thighs. • Press all the knuckles of your hands firmly into the floor to lift your chest higher to the ceiling. • Roll your shoulder blades toward each other. • Lift your belly in toward your spine.
• Lengthen the top of your head toward the ceiling.

GAZE & FOCUS Keep your gaze level with your head and look at a spot on the wall in front of you. • The only contact points with the floor are your hands and feet.

Press firmly into your foundation and lift your chest so your shoulder blades squeeze in toward your spine.

DEEPEN Lift your gaze toward the ceiling.

COMMON CHALLENGES Lower back pain can prevent you from taking the pose without pain.

MODIFICATION Substitute with Low Cobra (see Strength Practice I for more details).

Sun Salutation B

Focus on your hands and feet, and keep your gaze steady and centered.

Chair, inhale with arms up (first round: hold for five breaths). • Forward Fold, exhale. • Halfway Lift, inhale. • Chaturanga, exhale. • Upward-Facing Dog, inhale. • Downward-Facing Dog, exhale. • Warrior 1, right side, inhale (first round: hold for five breaths). • Chaturanga, exhale. • Upward-Facing Dog, inhale. • Downward-Facing Dog, exhale. • Warrior 1, Left side, inhale (first round: hold for five breaths). • Chaturanga, exhale. • Upward-Facing Dog, inhale. • Downward-Facing Dog, exhale, stay for five breaths. • Step or jump forward. • Halfway Lift, inhale. • Forward Fold, exhale. • Chair, inhale. • Repeat for two more rounds. End with a Forward Fold.

NEW POSES FOR SUN SALUTATION B

Warrior 1

Warrior 1 opens and strengthens your ankles and hip flexors and builds your hamstring strength. (See photo on p. 106.)

SETUP From Downward-Facing Dog, step your right foot next to your right thumb. Spin your left heel down and ground it into the mat. Lift your arms up.

ALIGNMENT Point your back foot out about 60 degrees. • Press the outer edge of your back foot into the mat to connect all four corners of your foot to the floor. • Align your feet so your heels are in one line. Point your front foot toward the front of your mat. Bend your front knee over your ankle. • Spin the hip of your back leg toward the front of your mat. You will feel an opening in your back hip flexor. • Lift your belly button in toward your spine. Squeeze your front ribs toward each other. • Soften your shoulders away from your ears, and squeeze your shoulder blades toward your spine. Reach your arms up and spread out your fingers.

GAZE & FOCUS Set your gaze on a wall in front of you. • Squeeze your back leg straight. Hug your core in and up toward your centerline.

DEEPEN Lengthen your stance and bend your front knee to a 90-degree angle.

MODIFICATIONS Shorten your stance slightly for both challenges until your ankle and hip flexors become more mobile. • Lift your back heel for a Crescent Lunge modification.

Chair

Chair requires powerful leg and core strength. Keep your shoulders engaged and palms facing inward to get used to rotating your shoulders down toward your spine. (See photo on p. 104.)

SETUP Stand with your feet together. Lower your hips toward the floor until you feel your legs engage. Keep your toes in view when you look at your knees. Reach your arms up, parallel to your ears with palms facing.

ALIGNMENT Keep your toes soft and in view just past your knees. • Spread out your toes. Lift your arches and spin your inner ankles toward the back of your mat. • Squeeze your inner thighs toward each other. • Tilt your tailbone toward the floor. Pull your belly in to activate your core. • Lift your chest over your hips and pull your front ribs together. • Soften your shoulders down away from your ears. Engage your back to pull your shoulder blades in toward each other. • Straighten your arms, stretch out your palms and spread your fingers wide toward the ceiling.

GAZE & FOCUS Set your drishti at a spot on the wall in front of you. • Focus on strength in your legs and a strong lift in your chest toward the ceiling.

DEEPEN Sink your hips deeper toward the floor. Keep your spine lifted toward the ceiling.

COMMON CHALLENGES Weak quadriceps may pull your knees away from each other. • Tight shoulders prevent you from bringing your arms overhead.

MODIFICATIONS Lift the arches of your feet to hug your knees toward each other. • Bend your elbows even with your shoulders at 90-degree angles like a cactus.

STRENGTH

Create more stability in your lower body by adding on new, challenging standing poses in this section of the practice.

Hand-to-Big-Toe Forward Fold

Active Forward Folds open your spine and create more space in your lower back. Harness your shoulders and back muscles to deepen your forward bend. In this Hand-to-Big-Toe Forward Fold pose, your big toes serve as an anchor for your hands to pull your chest deeper into the fold, opening your lower back and your hamstrings. Keep your knees bent, particularly if your hamstrings feel tight in general or from an active day on the wall.

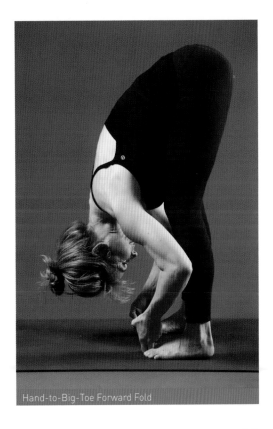
Hand-to-Big-Toe Forward Fold

SETUP Stack your feet directly under your hips—place two fists between your feet to measure. Loop your peace fingers (index and middle finger) around your big toes. Pull up on your big toes and press the four corners of your feet down toward the floor.

ALIGNMENT Bend your elbows to the outer edges of your mat to pull your chest toward your shins. • Hug your shoulder blades toward your spine. Engage the muscles under your shoulders to go deeper into the pose. • Bend your knees as needed—don't lock them!—and bring your belly down to your thighs. Squeeze your thighs. • Release your head toward the floor.

GAZE & FOCUS Look at the floor between your feet. • Squeeze your shoulder blades toward your spine to pull your chest closer toward your feet.

DEEPEN Work your legs as straight as your hamstrings allow while hugging your thigh muscles; do not force your legs to straighten and keep your knee joints soft.

SEQUENCE TRANSITION Release your big toes.

Gorilla

A big wrist and hand release, Gorilla is a counter pose to Plank, Chaturanga, and Downward-Facing Dog. It releases the impact of weight bearing in your wrists, which is important when you spend much of your time gripping holds. Do both hand variations to open your wrists and palms in two directions and free your hands to stretch completely.

SETUP Stand with your feet at hip-width distance. Bend your knees. Slide your hands underneath your feet, palms facing up and fingers reaching toward your heels.

ALIGNMENT Wiggle your hands deeper under your feet until your toes reach your wrists. • Bend your elbows to the outer edges of your mat. • Hug your shoulder blades together. Use your big trunk muscles under your shoulders to pull your chest deeper toward your spine. • Soften your knees and bring your belly down to your thighs. Engage your thigh muscles. • Release your neck and hang your head toward the floor.

GORILLA VARIATION Flip your hands so your palms face the floor with your fingers pointing in toward your heels, thumbs toward the outer edges of your feet. Slide your hands under your feet as deeply as you can go. Bend your elbows and soften your knees.

GAZE & FOCUS Look at the floor behind your feet. • Engage your shoulders and back muscles to pull your chest closer to your shins.

DEEPEN Work your legs as straight as your hamstrings allow while still squeezing your thighs. Keep your knee joints soft.

COMMON CHALLENGES Tight hamstrings prevent you from sliding your hands under your feet.

MODIFICATION Make fists and place the tops of your hands on a block, curled fingers facing in toward your body. Bend your knees.

SEQUENCE TRANSITION Release your hands from under your feet. • Bring your feet together. • Stand in Mountain Pose.

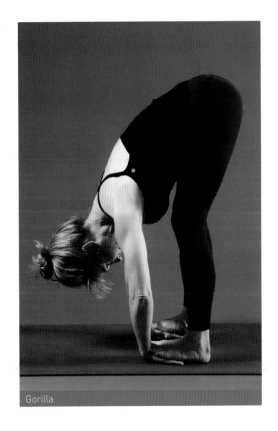
Gorilla

Twisted Chair

Focus on the alignment in Twisted Chair to better understand where your hips are in space while rotating your spine—a useful skill for climbing moves that require you to twist!

SETUP Bring your toes together and lower your hips into Chair. Connect your palms together in front of your chest. • On your exhale, twist to the left, hooking your right elbow outside your left knee.

ALIGNMENT Soften your toes and ground the four corners of your feet into the floor. • Make sure your knees stay even; knees askew are an indicator you are popping out a hip to one side. • Lift your left elbow up to the ceiling; press through your hands to deepen your twist. • Pull your belly in toward your spine and stick your sit bones out behind you. • Stretch your chest and head forward, pulling your shoulder blades toward your spine. • Open your lower hand to a block just outside your left foot. Extend your upper hand to the ceiling, palm facing the same direction as your chest.

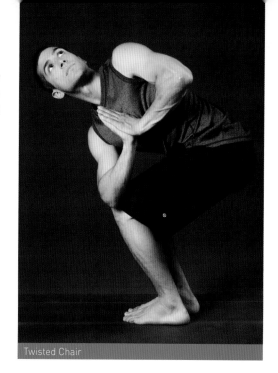

Twisted Chair

GAZE & FOCUS Look up at the ceiling past your upper hand. • Keep your knees even and aligned throughout the twist.

DEEPEN Settle your hips lower toward the floor. Hug your inner thighs toward each other and rotate your upper ribs to the ceiling.

COMMON CHALLENGES A lack of torso rotation prevents you from reaching your lower hand to the outside edge of your foot.

MODIFICATION Bring the block just in front of your feet to support the extension in your twist.

SEQUENCE TRANSITION Release your chest forward to your feet. • Inhale and lengthen your chest to Halfway Lift. • Step your left foot to the back of your mat.

Crescent Lunge

A great stabilizing pose, Crescent Lunge develops the muscles around your front knee, and strengthens your thighs, hamstrings, and glutes even more than the Low Lunge. Here, you learn to stabilize into the centerline by hugging your inner thighs to your pelvis and engaging your core.

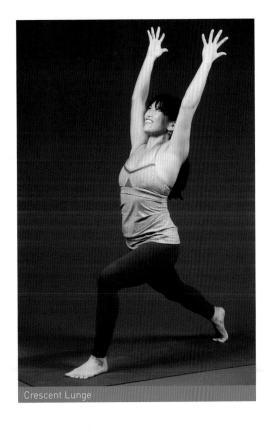

Crescent Lunge

SETUP From a lunge position in your legs, stack your front knee over your ankle. Lift onto the ball of your left foot, toes bent, so your left heel is perpendicular to the ground. Squeeze your back hamstring straight. • Lift your chest over your hips and extend your arms straight up to the ceiling.

ALIGNMENT Move your feet hip-width distance apart for stability. Press your front foot into the ground. • Lift your back hamstring up to the ceiling. • Square your pelvis toward the front of your mat. Squeeze your front heel and back foot toward each other. • Pull in your core lock. • Release your shoulders away from your ears. Reach your arms up to the ceiling parallel to your ears, pinky fingers forward. • Pull your shoulder blades in toward each other.

GAZE & FOCUS Set your drishti at a spot on the wall in front of you. • Ground your front foot and straighten your back leg.

DEEPEN Lengthen your stance and bend your front knee to a 90-degree angle.

COMMON CHALLENGES Your front foot moves around.

MODIFICATIONS Ground into the big toe knuckle at the base of your front foot, and your heel. Lower your back knee to the floor for a Low Lunge if you need to.

Twisted Crescent Lunge

Adding a twist to an already challenging standing pose requires your body to stabilize to hold the pose. Twists create a healthy opening for your spine and release tightness that has accumulated in your lower back and shoulders from climbing. Your glutes also will activate.

SETUP From Crescent Lunge, bring your palms together in front of your chest. On your exhale, hook your right elbow outside your left knee.

ALIGNMENT Squeeze your feet in toward each other to activate your inner thighs and stabilize your legs. Keep your front knee stacked over your ankle. • Squeeze your back thigh muscles, and straighten your back leg toward the ceiling. • Lift your upper elbow toward the ceiling. Press down into both palms equally. • Hug your belly in toward your spine, elevating your front ribs off your front thigh. • Pull your shoulders in toward your chest, and lengthen your chest forward to keep your spine long and straight and to deepen your twist. • Keep your shoulders higher than your hips.

GAZE & FOCUS Set your gaze on a spot on the ceiling. • Squeeze your shoulder blades toward each other. Engage the muscles underneath your shoulder blades to deepen your twist.

DEEPEN Open your arms, with your lower hand on the floor or on a block outside your front leg. Lift your upper hand to the ceiling, palm facing the same direction as your chest. • Stretch your upper fingers away from your body.

COMMON CHALLENGES You will need to develop strength and stability in your legs to hold the full pose. Squeeze your inner thighs for balance.

MODIFICATION Keep your back knee on the floor. Pad your knee if you feel pain in your kneecap.

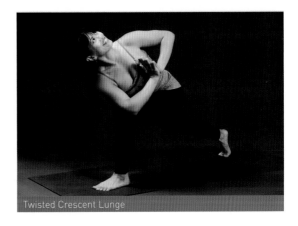
Twisted Crescent Lunge

SEQUENCE TRANSITION Release your hands to the floor. • Ground your back heel, and lift your torso above your hips for Warrior 2.

Warrior 2

Widen your stance and bend your front knee deeper to challenge yourself in your evolving Warrior 2. Practice bringing ease into your face and your experience of the pose, and imagine bringing the same softness to solving a problem on a climb.

SETUP On an exhale, ground your back heel to the mat. Stack your chest over your hips and extend your arms. Open your back toes so your foot is parallel with the back edge of your mat. Bend your front knee over your front ankle; don't let your knee cave in. Stretch your arms toward the front and back parallel with the floor, and set your gaze over your front hand.

ALIGNMENT Point your front foot toward the front of your mat. Stack your front knee over your ankle. (Widen your feet if your knee is bending past the top of your ankle.) • Line your back foot up with the back edge of your mat at roughly 90 degrees, but no wider than that, from your front foot. Lift the inner arch of your back foot off the floor. • Hug your feet toward each other to activate your inner thighs toward your pelvis. • Press your front heel firmly into the mat. • Stack your chest over your hips. Lengthen your tailbone down toward the floor. Lift your belly button in toward your spine. • Release your shoulders away from your ears. Hover your arms parallel to the floor. • Pull your shoulders in toward your centerline. From your spine, stretch your fingers to the front and back walls.

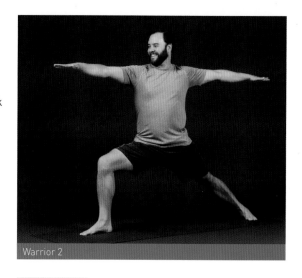

Warrior 2

GAZE & FOCUS Turn your head toward your front hand and set your gaze on your fingertips.
• Squeeze your thigh bones in toward each other. Relax your jaw and eyes. Breathe into the challenge.

DEEPEN Widen your stance and bend your right thigh parallel to the floor.

COMMON CHALLENGES Weak or tight outer hips and glutes can cause your front knee to collapse inward rather than staying stacked over your front ankle.

MODIFICATIONS Shorten your stance. Keep your knee aligned over your front ankle to build strength and prevent injury.

SEQUENCE TRANSITION From Warrior 2, straighten your front leg.

Triangle

A pose to ground you, Triangle relies on your bone structure rather than muscle strength to bring attention to your hamstrings, hips, and spine. Challenge your stability and see what is possible in the pose with a longer stance.

SETUP With both legs straight, reach your front hand toward the front of your mat until your torso is parallel to the floor. Shift your front hip toward the back of your mat. Place your right hand on your front shin or on a block outside your right foot. Reach your upper hand toward the ceiling.

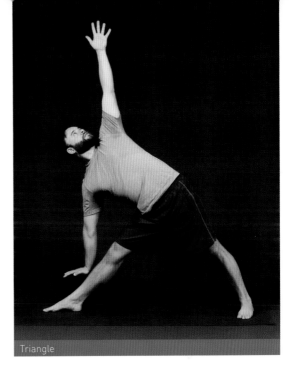

Triangle

ALIGNMENT Ground the four corners of both feet into the floor. • Pull your front thigh bone up into your hip socket; your back hip will roll slightly forward toward the floor. • Lift the top of your right kneecap to contract your thigh muscle. Keep a slight bend in your front knee so you don't lock or hyperextend into the joint. • Hug your shoulders in toward your spine. • Stretch your chest toward the front of your mat; spin your upper ribs toward the ceiling. • Stretch out your fingers on your upper hand.

GAZE & FOCUS Look up at the ceiling and set your gaze on one spot. • Press your big toe knuckle of your front foot into the floor. Focus on the stability of your legs and length in your spine.

DEEPEN Widen your stance. Reach your lower hand deeper toward your ankle or the floor.

COMMON CHALLENGES Tight hamstrings or a tight psoas prevent you from reaching your shin. • You overextend in your front knee joint.

MODIFICATION Use a block at the tallest height outside your front foot. If necessary, stack two blocks to get enough height to lengthen your spine. • Soften

your front knee joint and lift the muscles above your knee.

SEQUENCE TRANSITION From Triangle on an inhale, lift your chest over your hips for Warrior 2.

Half-Bound Side Angle

Open your tight climbing shoulders with a half bind in your Side Angle. In addition to the challenge of holding the pose in your legs, you also can release in your upper shoulder and neck through the bind. It's a glorious, intense release.

SETUP From Warrior 2, bring your front hand to a block inside your front foot. Hug your outer right hip toward your back foot. Reach your upper arm to the ceiling, then wind the top of your hand around your lower back. Walk your fingers in toward your front inner thigh for the bind. If you can't reach your thigh, grab some clothing.

ALIGNMENT Ground the four corners of both feet into the floor. Squeeze both feet toward the center

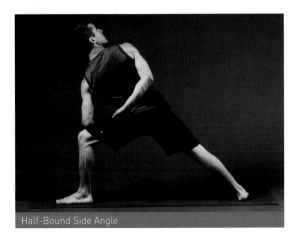
Half-Bound Side Angle

front inner thigh. • Pull your belly in toward your spine.• Lengthen the crown of your head and spiral your chest toward the ceiling. Notice the release in your neck.

GAZE & FOCUS Set your gaze on the ceiling.
• Breathe into your upper shoulder as it releases through the bind.

DEEPEN Reach your lower hand under your front thigh and clasp your bound hand to create a full bind. • Move your hands toward your front knee and lift your chest off your thigh.

COMMON CHALLENGES Weak glutes cause your front knee to collapse inward.

MODIFICATION Shorten your stance slightly as long as you keep your front knee aligned over your ankle.

SEQUENCE TRANSITION Stretch your upper arm to the ceiling to release. • Lift your chest to Warrior 2.
• Straighten your front leg. • Turn your right foot to left edge of your mat so your feet are parallel.

of your mat. • Stack your front knee over your front ankle. • Pull your front thigh bone into your hip socket until you feel your outer glute engage.
• Keep your right hip even with your bent front knee.
• Lift the arch of your back foot and squeeze your back inner thigh. • Engage your belly to lighten the weight of your front arm on your thigh. • Roll the top of your upper shoulder in toward your chest. Walk your fingers deeper into the bind toward your

Wide-Legged Forward Fold

This pose reaches deeply into new regions of your hamstrings and inner thighs—creating more space in your spine. Legs that work hard balancing on a wall will appreciate this pose.

SETUP With your feet parallel to each other, widen your heels just outside your toes until the outer edges of your feet are parallel to the mat. Bring your hands to your hips. On an inhale, lift your chest to the ceiling; on an exhale, fold forward.

ALIGNMENT Bring your hands to the floor under your shoulders. Point your fingers in the same direction as your toes. • If your hamstrings and lower back allow, walk your hands back between your feet. • Lift the arches of your feet; squeeze your inner thighs up toward your pelvis. • Pull your chest deeper toward the floor with your hands.
• **Left side:** Interlace your hands at your lower back. Hug your shoulder blades in toward your spine. Straighten your arms, press your hands away from your lower back and fold forward.

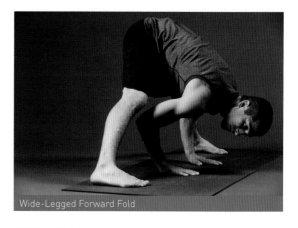

Wide-Legged Forward Fold

GAZE & FOCUS Look at a spot on your mat between your feet; resist the urge to look around! • Squeeze your thigh muscles and shift your weight slightly forward toward your toes.

DEEPEN Straighten your legs. Pull your head toward your mat.

COMMON CHALLENGES Tight hamstrings or lower back prevent your hands from reaching the floor.

MODIFICATION Use a block under your hands. Bend your knees to give your spine more space.

TRIPOD HEADSTAND VARIATION Bring the crown of your head—the spot between your forehead and the top of your head—to the floor. Walk your wrists back so you have a triangular base between your hands and your head. Stack your elbows over your wrists. Hug your elbows in toward each other. When your arms feel stable, engage your core. • If you are new to Tripod, practice the Variation in Crow (see later in the chapter.) If you are stable in Tripod, slowly lift your feet from the wide-legged position until they are stacked over your head. Squeeze your core throughout the headstand.

SEQUENCE TRANSITION From the fold, walk your hands forward underneath your shoulders. • Turn your toes on your back foot out at a slight angle, and bend your back knee for Skandasana.

Skandasana

Moving your body in different planes of motion is inherent to climbing. Skandasana adds in a side-to-side movement to your practice, and strengthens legs and hips. A deep side lunge, it is particularly effective for refining balance and practicing rotating your hips and spine in different directions.

SETUP Bend your back knee over your back foot, keeping your heel on the ground. Ground your front foot into the mat.

ALIGNMENT Deepen into the lunge toward your back foot. Keep your front foot parallel. • Lift the arches of your feet off the floor and pull your feet in toward each other. • Stack your hands underneath your shoulders. Lengthen your chest parallel with your hips. Widen your sit bones out behind you. • Lift your front ribs into your body. • Engage your inner thighs toward your pelvis. • Hug your shoulders into your back, and engage your core.

VARIATION Turn your back toes out to a 45-degree angle, and bend your knee even deeper with your back heel *still grounded*. Flex your front toes up to the sky, your heel on the ground. • Bring both hands together, pressing your left elbow into your inner knee.

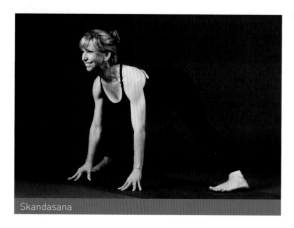
Skandasana

GAZE & FOCUS Look at one spot on the floor directly at a natural point between your hands. • Play with the bend in your knee and keep your core engaged.

COMMON CHALLENGES Tight hips and lower back prevent your hands from reaching the floor.

MODIFICATIONS Stay in the first variation of the pose with feet flat on your mat. Stack your hands under your shoulders on a block.

SEQUENCE TRANSITION Straighten your back leg. • Walk your hands back to the front edge of your mat. • Step your back foot to meet your front foot. Bring your feet together and do a Halfway Lift, inhale. • Exhale and Forward Fold. • Complete the sequence from Twisted Chair through Skandasana on your left side. • Step to the front edge of your mat.

Squat

A squat releases your lower back and hips, and allows your body to move into the natural curves of your spine. It also opens your ankles. Activate your feet, press your elbows into your knees, and work on lifting your chest to release your spine.

SETUP Walk your feet as wide as your mat. Bend your knees to lower your hips toward the floor. If your heels lift off the floor, widen your stance until you can get your feet flat. Your toes can turn out wider than your heels. • Bring your hands together, palms touching, in front of your chest.

ALIGNMENT Shift your weight into the outer arches of your feet, and lift your inner arches. Squeeze your

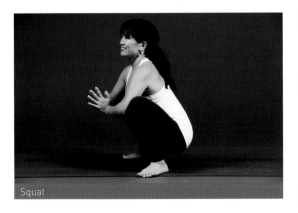
Squat

DEEPEN Bring your feet wider and sink your tailbone closer toward the floor. Work your feet toward parallel.

COMMON CHALLENGES Tight hips prevent you from grounding your heels.

MODIFICATION If you have trouble lowering down below your knees, stay in a higher squat position or bring a folded blanket under your heels.

Crow

heels in toward each other like you are trying to wrinkle your mat. • Lift your belly button in toward your spine to lift your chest toward the ceiling. • Press your elbows into your inner knees. • Stay for ten breaths.

GAZE & FOCUS Set your gaze on a spot on the wall ahead. • Lengthen your spine and keep your knees aligned over your feet. • Play with sitting in a passive squat, then engage your pelvic floor and lift your hips an inch out of the bottom of the squat into an active one.

Crow is yoga wrapped up into one tiny arm balance. It presents mental and physical challenges all at once. I have heard every reason possible why people can't do this pose—my arms aren't strong enough, I'm scared to fall over, what's the point of this pose? The point is to trust yourself and learn to do something that scares you—a whole new world of possibilities awaits.

SETUP From a Squat, set your hands on the floor a foot in front of you so your hands are underneath your shoulders. Lift your hips until your shoulders come over your wrists and your hips are shoulder height or higher. • Lift your hips above your shoulders, and walk your feet in closer toward each other. Bend your elbows slightly and wrap them back toward parallel. Place your knees on your upper arms above your elbows. • Shift your weight forward to take all your weight into your arms.

ALIGNMENT Keep your gaze forward in front of your hands for balance. • Put all your weight into your hands. Lift one foot off the floor. Try the other foot. • If you can balance with one foot off the floor, slowly lift the other one. • Safety note: Do not hop into the pose. Move mindfully, leaning your weight into your arms with your gaze lifted so your head can counterbalance the weight of your body. • Lift your feet slowly. • Release into a Squat.

GAZE & FOCUS Lift your drishti to the floor past your fingertips. • Play with transferring your weight into your hands, with your head and gaze still lifted forward.

DEEPEN Bring your big toes together while hovering off the floor in the pose. Straighten your arms.

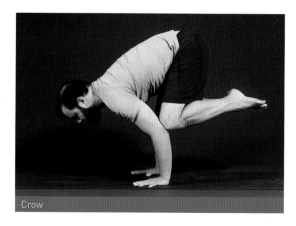

Crow

TRIPOD HEADSTAND VARIATION Lower the crown of your head—the spot between the top of your head and hairline—to the floor in front of your hands. • Make sure your hands and head are in a stable triangle shape. Wrap your elbows toward each other and pull your shoulders into your back. • Your knees still should be on your upper arms. Tilt your hips forward until they are stacked above your shoulders and slowly pull one knee in toward your chest. If you are stable, pull your other knee in toward your chest. • Hold with your knees in at your chest, and squeeze into your centerline. • If you are stable, extend one leg at a time toward the ceiling. Flex your feet. If you feel unstable, bring your feet down or practice somersaulting out. Only take this pose if you feel comfortable rolling out. Leave yourself room! • Note: When new to inversions, you can also practice against a wall until you are comfortable trying this in the middle of the room.

COMMON CHALLENGES If you have a wrist injury, be mindful in Crow.

MODIFICATION Squat with your heels on the floor.

SEQUENCE TRANSITION From a Squat, lift your hips up to the sky into a Forward Fold. • Walk your big toes to touch. • Inhale and reach your arms up to the sky.

Eagle

Observe if your shoulders are starting to open in the bind and focus on breathing deeply into the sensations. Set your gaze and bend your standing leg more deeply for more challenge.

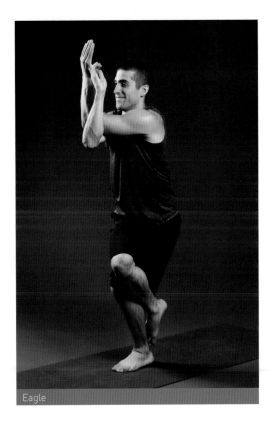

Eagle

SETUP From Mountain Pose, extend your arms out wide and parallel to the floor, palms facing forward. Cross your right upper arm underneath your left upper arm. Wind your forearms around each other. Bring your palms to touch for the full bind. • Lower into Chair in your legs. Cross your right thigh on top of your left thigh.

ALIGNMENT Ground into your standing foot. Squeeze your inner thighs all the way together. • Stretch out your toes on your upper foot. • Stack your shoulders over your hips; engage your core lock. • Lift your elbows level with your shoulders. Press your hands away from your face to stack your wrists over your elbows. • Soften your shoulders away from your ears; pull your arm bones in toward your shoulder sockets.

GAZE & FOCUS Look past your arms to a spot on the wall. • Engage your belly firmly and set your gaze.

DEEPEN Bend your standing leg deeper and wrap your right foot around your calf. Challenge your balance by moving your gaze in toward your forearms.

COMMON CHALLENGES Tight shoulders can prevent you from taking a full bind.

MODIFICATION Reach for opposite shoulders and lift your elbows even with your shoulders.

SEQUENCE TRANSITION Release to Mountain Pose. • Do Eagle on the left side; wrap your left arm under your right and lift your left leg over your right leg.

Hand-to-Knee Balancing Pose

Your body relies on several systems for balance, including feet, core, and gaze. Hand-to-Knee Balancing pose challenges your balance by using your standing leg as the foundation while your other leg switches positions and directions. You also move your gaze, testing your inner ear balance and eyes. It's a poetic little series of poses.

SETUP Stand in Mountain Pose. Ground into the four corners of your left foot. Lift your right knee even with your hip and hold your knee with your right hand.

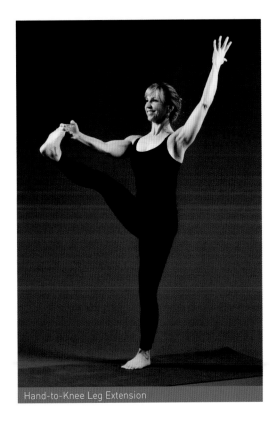

Hand-to-Knee Leg Extension

ALIGNMENT Hug your belly in toward your spine.
• Extend your free arm up to the ceiling, palm facing your body. • Lower your shoulders away from your ears and pull your shoulder blades toward each other. • Stay for five breaths.

GAZE Look at a spot on the wall in front of you.

DEEPEN Loop your peace fingers around your big toe. Extend your leg forward for a balance challenge and hamstring opening. Squeeze your right thigh muscles to lengthen your hamstring. Maintaining a long, neutral spine is more important than the extension. Focus on standing up straight. Pull the shoulder of your extended arm in toward your spine. Lengthen your leg last.

HAND-TO-KNEE SIDE On an inhale, move your knee to the right. Extend your left hand toward the opposite side of the room, palm facing up. • Pull your right thigh bone into your hip socket to keep your pelvis level and your leg integrated into your body. • Lower your shoulders down your back and squeeze your shoulder blades toward each other. • Stay for five

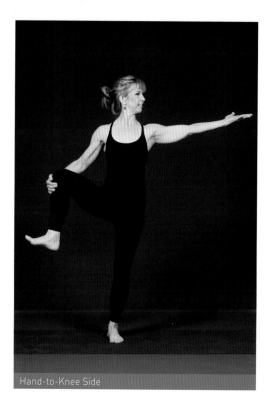
Hand-to-Knee Side

breaths. • **Gaze:** Move your gaze over your left palm. • **Deepen:** While holding your big toe, open your leg to the right. Hug your right thighbone into your hip socket to keep your pelvis level and spin your inner right thigh up to the ceiling. The tendency is to lose the centerline, which makes the balance harder! Press through your lifted heel and hug your thigh muscles to the bone.

HAND-TO-KNEE LEG EXTENSION On an inhale, bring your right leg back knee back in front of you. Extend your right leg forward and parallel with the floor. • Press through your extended heel. Lift your arms straight up to the ceiling. • Stack your shoulders over your hips. Engage your core. If you feel it in your lower back, you are leaning back too far. • Engage your shoulders toward each other. • Set your drishti at your extended foot. • Stay for five breaths.

SEQUENCE TRANSITION Release your upper foot and stand in Mountain Pose. • Do all the Hand-to-Knee variations on your left side. • Come to stand in Mountain Pose.

Airplane

As the name implies, this pose benefits from a lift in your chest like the nose of an airplane. Your standing leg becomes a lever, and the lean of your chest counterbalances the lift of your leg behind you, developing great functional strength for understanding balance no matter the circumstances while climbing. Activate your core to support your lower back.

SETUP Stand tall in Mountain Pose. Shift your weight to your left foot. Extend your right foot toward the back of your mat. Reach your hands back toward your legs and float them above your hips.

ALIGNMENT Flex the toes on your back foot toward your kneecap. • Lift your shoulders just above your hips. • Hug your shoulder blades onto your spine. Rotate your thumbs away from your body, with your palms facing down. • Rotate your right hip down and level with your left hip so your toes point toward the floor. Pull your right thigh bone into your hip socket. • Engage your core lock. • Elevate your right foot even with your head.

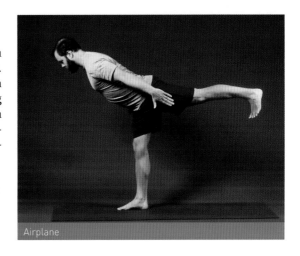

Airplane

GAZE & FOCUS Look at the floor in front of your standing foot. • Lift your back leg until you feel your hamstrings engage. Keep your belly lifted in and up.

DEEPEN Extend your arms forward and parallel with your head to take the pose to Warrior 3.

COMMON CHALLENGES A lack of strength and balance challenges you to stay steady in the pose.

MODIFICATIONS Bring your hands to a block placed directly under each of your shoulders to balance. Lift your chest and engage your back muscles and core. • Extend your back leg parallel with the floor.

SEQUENCE TRANSITION In Airplane, bring your hands together at your chest. • Lower your left hand to a block just to the left of your left foot. • Roll your right hip open for Half Moon.

Half Moon

Another balancing pose, Half Moon requires engagement in your standing leg and strength in your glutes. Practice this pose and you will have a deeper understanding of your strength and grace in the pose and while flowing into moves on the wall.

SETUP Line up a block (at its tallest height) underneath your left shoulder, just to the left of your standing pinky toe. Bring your left hand to the block. Shift your weight into your left foot. • Lift your right leg and roll your right hip on top of your left. Lift your upper arm to the ceiling.

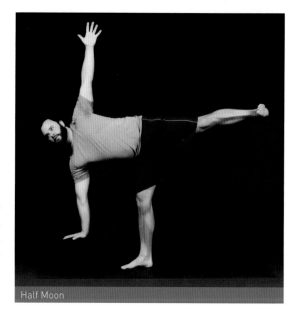
Half Moon

ALIGNMENT Press firmly into your standing foot with your toes pointing straight forward. Squeeze your thighs. • Flex the toes of your lifted leg. Bring your lifted leg in line with your hip. You should be able to see your back toes. • Pull your upper thigh bone in toward your hip. Notice your upper glute engage; lift your upper leg higher. • Extend your chest long, pulling your belly in toward your spine. • Keep the weight on your lower hand light; rely on your standing leg for strength. • Pull your shoulder blades into your back. Extend your upper fingers to the ceiling.

GAZE & FOCUS Look at the floor. • Press deeply into your standing foot and radiate out from your core in every direction.

DEEPEN Move your gaze to the ceiling. Lighten the touch of your lower hand on the block or floor.

COMMON CHALLENGES You have trouble balancing in the middle of the room.

MODIFICATION Do this pose against a wall for support.

SEQUENCE TRANSITION Bring both hands to the floor. • Step your upper leg about halfway back on your mat for Revolved Triangle.

Revolved Triangle

A twist and a balance rolled up into one pose, Revolved Triangle can sometimes feel like patting your head and rubbing your belly at the same time. It requires stability in your legs to free your spine for the twist. Like a crux climbing move that requires your body to move in multiple directions, the pose will test your body awareness, determination, and focus.

SETUP Set your feet up in a stance slightly shorter than Warrior 1 (the distance between your front and back foot is about the length of your leg). Take your feet about hip-width distance, back foot set at about a 45-degree angle, for lateral stability. Take your left hand to your left hip. • Stand up and extend your right arm up to the ceiling. Lower your chest parallel to the floor, your core lock engaged. • Bring your right hand to a block at the tallest or middle height inside your front shin.

ALIGNMENT Press your back foot into the floor and lengthen your tailbone to press your sit bones

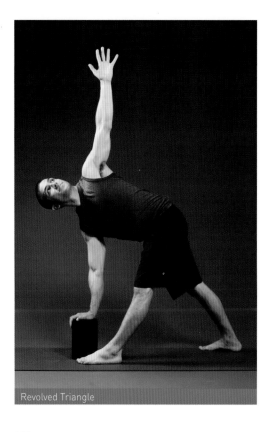

Revolved Triangle

to the wall behind you. • Distribute your weight evenly between front and back foot. • Squeeze your thigh muscles, including your inner thighs, toward your pelvis. • Pull your belly in toward your spine. • Stretch your chest parallel to the floor to lengthen your spine. • With your left hand still on your hip, squeeze your shoulder blades in toward your spine and spin your chest left and up toward the ceiling. • Reach your left arm up to the ceiling.

GAZE & FOCUS Look at your upper hand. • Press your back foot deeply into the mat. Rotate from your oblique muscles.

DEEPEN Bring your lower hand to the floor inside your foot, or place your block outside your front foot to challenge your balance and twist.

COMMON CHALLENGES Weak glutes or tight hamstrings prevent you from grounding your back foot and keeping your hips even as you twist.

MODIFICATIONS Use the block at the tallest height or even your shin, avoiding your knee. Focus on grounding your feet before you twist.

Step to the front edge of your mat. Complete Airplane, Half Moon, and Revolved Triangle on your left side. • Bring your hands to the floor for Plank. • Lower to Chaturanga, exhale.
• Lift your chest to Upward-Facing Dog, inhale.
• Exhale into Downward-Facing Dog.

BACKBENDS

A backbend practice ramps up the intensity, moving you even deeper into your spine and opening your shoulders, particularly when you add in a Wheel. Build upon what you have learned about opening your chest, engaging your big back muscles, and learn to activate the smaller muscles around your spine to work safely into your backbends.

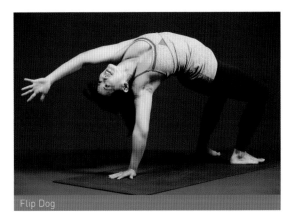
Flip Dog

Flip Dog

Bring lightness and flow into your Flip Dog, landing quietly into the pose and exiting with energy when you hop back over.

SETUP From Downward-Facing Dog, lift your right leg to the ceiling. Bend your right knee and roll your hip open for Three-Legged Dog. • Look under your left arm for your upper foot and lower it to the floor behind you. Turn your other foot around 180 degrees until both toes are flat and parallel on the ground.
• Keep your left hand where it started on the ground and reach your free arm overhead toward the floor.

ALIGNMENT Set your feet hip-width distance.
• Press into the four corners of your feet and lift

your hips to the ceiling. • Bend your right elbow even with your shoulder for a cactus arm. Hug your shoulder blades toward each other to open your chest. • Engage your core lock. • Soften your neck to let your head hang toward the floor.

GAZE & FOCUS Set your gaze on the front wall or the floor under you. • Press down into your feet to lift your hips higher. Hug your shoulder blades in toward your spine.

DEEPEN Reach your hand overhead toward the floor.

COMMON CHALLENGES If you have shoulder pain, be mindful in this pose—and skip if it exacerbates the injury.

MODIFICATION Stay in Three-Legged Dog.

SEQUENCE TRANSITION To release, lift your right arm to the ceiling. • Hop back over to Three-Legged Dog. • Lower your upper foot and move forward to Plank. • Bring your feet together, shift your weight into your right hand, and roll to the outer edge of your right foot.

Side Plank

The more you practice rotating your shoulders away from your chest toward your spine, the more natural it will feel. When you add your own body weight, it balances your shoulder strength and keeps a heavily used joint healthy for more climbing.

SETUP Stack your left foot on top of your right foot. Move your right shoulder over your right wrist. Lift your left hand up to the ceiling, palm facing the same direction as your chest.

ALIGNMENT Your right fingers face the front of the mat and your right hand is stacked a couple of inches forward of your shoulder. • Flex your toes toward your knees and squeeze the muscles of your legs to the bone. • Keep your body at one angled plane from shoulders to feet. • Pull your shoulder blades in toward your spine to take the weight out of your wrist. • Spread out the fingers on your upper hand. • Lengthen the crown of your head toward the front of your mat.

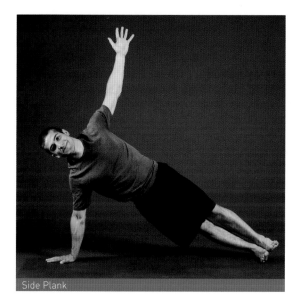
Side Plank

GAZE & FOCUS Look at the ceiling. • Create stability through your legs and core.

DEEPEN Lift your upper leg as high as you can toward the ceiling.

COMMON CHALLENGES You are still building strength and struggle to hold the pose.

MODIFICATION Bring your lower knee to the floor underneath your hip for support, keeping your foundation hand, lower knee and feet in one line.

SEQUENCE TRANSITION From Side Plank, lower your upper hand for Plank. • Roll forward on your toes and lower to Chaturanga. • Inhale and lift your chest to Upward-Facing Dog. • Exhale and lift your hips for Downward-Facing Dog. • Do Flip Dog to Side Plank on the left side. • Move forward to Plank and lower to the floor.

Locust

An active backbend, Locust builds strength in your lower back and activates the muscles around your spine. Your body must lift to counter gravity, strengthening to extend your chest and legs. Think about lifting from the front side of your body. It is a heart opener, after all.

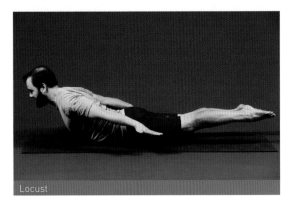
Locust

SETUP On your belly, bring your feet to hip-width distance, toes pointed. Reach your arms alongside your body, hands down by your hips, palms facing down.

ALIGNMENT Press the tops of your feet into the floor, and lift your knees off the ground. • Keep your upper legs engaged, and lift them off the floor. • Lengthen the crown of your head forward, and lengthen and lift your chest to the ceiling. Hug your shoulders in toward your spine. • Lift your upper arm bones toward the ceiling and float your hands above your hips. • Pull your belly up and in to lift even higher into the pose.

BOUND VARIATION Interlace your hands at your lower back. If you have tight shoulders and cannot do the bind, hold a strap with your hands to modify. Lift your hands off your lower back in the pose.

GAZE & FOCUS Look past your nose at the front edge of your mat or the floor. • Squeeze your legs, engage your core, and lift from your chest forward and up to the sky.

DEEPEN Bring your inner thighs and ankles together and lift.

COMMON CHALLENGES You feel lower back strain.

MODIFICATION Keep the tops of your feet on the floor. Place your hands by your lower ribs. • Lift your chest into Low Cobra.

SEQUENCE TRANSITION Do a second Locust with the Bound Variation. • Release to the floor.

A HEALTHY SPINE

Reversing your hunch from sitting at a computer all day takes practice—in case you missed that memo. Backbends are an effective way to signal to your brain that you want to open your chest, loosen your tight shoulders, and strengthen your lower back, which are all impacted from rolling your shoulders forward all day, a pattern that often continues when climbing.

The belly backbend Locust, for example, strengthens the muscles that arch your back, including the muscles along your spine, your lower back muscles, and your butt muscles. Upward-Facing Dog strengthens your arms in addition to opening your chest. Wheel, the deepest extension of the backbends, stretches deeply into your shoulders.

When first practicing backbends, most people tend to bend at the weakest point in their spine, particularly if their body is already open. Focus on keeping your core engaged, lengthening your lower back, and using your back strength to create a long, beautiful arc in your backbend.

Deep backbends foster healthy alignment, teach you to use your legs to access your core, strengthen and support your spine, and open your chest. Energetically, backbends also open your heart, and give you a path to connect to your body and energy. Instead of skipping them, learn to love them!

Bow

Strong legs are instrumental to backbends, and Bow pose teaches your body how to engage your legs for backbends, in addition to opening up your quadriceps and strengthening your back. It also is a powerful opening in your chest and shoulders.

SETUP From your belly on the floor, bend both knees. Reach for the outer edges of your feet with your hands.

ALIGNMENT Bring your knees to hip-width distance to support your lower back and tap into your leg strength. • Stretch out your toes and spin your inner

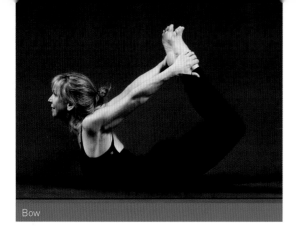
Bow

COMMON CHALLENGES Tight hamstrings or knee injuries prevent you from grabbing both of your feet at the same time.

MODIFICATION Bring your left forearm parallel to the front edge of your mat. Stack your left elbow under your left shoulder, palm facing down on the floor. Reach your right hand to your right foot. Press into your left elbow and lift your right foot up to the ceiling. • Do both sides. • Alternative: Substitute with Locust pose.

SEQUENCE TRANSITION Release your feet from Bow with care to the floor. • Press up to your hands and knees. • Move over to a seated position. • Set your feet hip-width distance and flat on the mat. • Lower down to your back.

ankles toward your lower back. • Pull your belly in toward your spine. • Press your pelvis down toward the floor. Lift your feet up toward the ceiling. • Use your leg strength to lift as high as you can.

GAZE & FOCUS Lift your eyes to the floor or the front of the room. • Engage your core and use your legs in the pose.

DEEPEN Reach for your ankles. Flex your toes and rock back to the tops of your thighs.

Bridge

Apply what you learned about leg strength in Bow for Bridge. The more you engage your legs, the stronger your backbends will be, opening your chest and shoulders.

SETUP Walk your feet closer to your body until your fingertips brush your heels. Set your feet parallel and hip-width distance. Press into the four corners of your feet to lift your hips to the ceiling. • Move your shoulders together and interlace your hands underneath your body.

ALIGNMENT Press your feet into your mat until your legs engage. • Stack your knees over your ankles. • Spin your inner thighs toward each other and down toward your mat. • Take one hand to your spine just above the tailbone. Feel the ridge of muscles around your spine engage. Lift your spine until you feel the engagement between your shoulder blades. • Lift your chest toward the back wall. • Squeeze your front ribs together.

GAZE & FOCUS Look at a spot on the ceiling. • Press deeply into your feet for strong legs.

DEEPEN Lift your right knee into your chest. Press strongly into your rooted foot. Extend your right leg, foot flexed, to the ceiling, keeping your hips level. Switch sides.

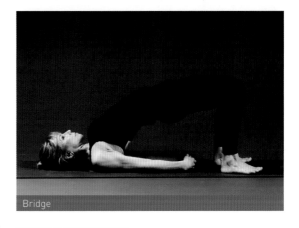

Bridge

COMMON CHALLENGES Tight shoulders prevent you from interlacing your hands.

MODIFICATION Use a strap between your hands for a bind. Or press your palms into the floor.

SEQUENCE TRANSITION To release, reach your arms up to the ceiling and slowly lower down the length of your spine. • Keep your feet in the Bridge setup to prepare for Wheel.

Wheel

Wheel is where all the alignment you have learned comes together. A fully extended backbend, this peak pose requires powerful legs, integrated shoulders, and deep breathing. You will experience strength, heart opening, and an energy burst. If the last time you did this pose was around the age of six, today is the best day to start.

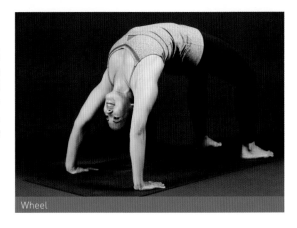

Wheel

SETUP From your Bridge with your feet at hip-width distance, plant your hands on either side of your head as wide as your mat, fingers turned in toward your shoulders. Point your elbows directly to the back of your mat. Lift your hips like you are going into Bridge. Push down into the floor with your hands. • Set the crown of your head on the floor and wrap your elbows in toward each other so your upper arms are parallel. Press your hands down into the floor to straighten your arms.

ALIGNMENT Ground your feet deeply into the floor. • Spiral your inner thighs toward each other and down toward your mat. • Pull your shoulders away from your ears, and wrap your shoulder blades in toward your spine. • Press your hands deeply into the earth. • Pull your front ribs in toward each other. • Tilt your tailbone and pull your pubic bone toward your ribs to lengthen your lower back. • Let your head hang toward the floor.

GAZE & FOCUS Look at the floor behind you. • Push into your feet to get strong in your legs. Spin your inner thighs toward each other and down toward the floor. Pull your shoulder blades in together.

DEEPEN Place a block between your inner thighs at the narrowest height as high as it will go. Come up to Wheel while squeezing the block.

COMMON CHALLENGES Shoulder or wrist injuries may prevent you from accessing the full pose. • You struggle to straighten your arms. • The pose puts pressure on your lower back.

MODIFICATION For shoulder or wrist injuries, stay in Bridge pose. • To create more space in your shoulders, place your hands as wide as your mat. • For lower back pain, bring your feet wider and spin your inner thighs toward the floor. Hug your belly in before you come up. If you are still feeling lower back pain, build strength in Bridge.

SEQUENCE TRANSITION To release, tuck your chin, lower to the back of your head, and slowly lower down the length of your spine. • Do Wheel three times total. • Come down to your back, and bring the bottoms of your feet together for Supine Butterfly. Stay for five breaths. • Rock up to a seated position. • Move to Downward-Facing Dog.

Lizard

A deep, dynamic hip opener, your hips may be more inclined to shout at you than sigh with delight here. Either way, Lizard is a release valve for your glutes and hips. Catch your back foot for a stretch deep into your quads while working toward a higher high step.

SETUP From Downward-Facing Dog, step your right foot outside your right hand. Lower your back knee to the mat.

ALIGNMENT Flex your front foot and roll to the outer edge of your foot. The sole of your foot is off the floor and your right knee will roll open. • Lower your elbows down beside your foot with elbows roughly in line with your heel. • Release your head toward your hands. • Stay for ten breaths.

GAZE & FOCUS Look at the floor just inside your front foot. • Notice the sensations in your hip and send your breath there.

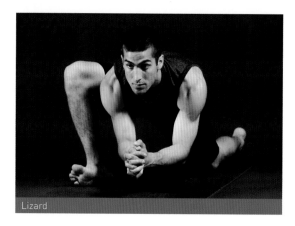

Lizard

DEEPEN Do not bind your Lizard. Instead, tuck your back toes, squeeze your quads, and lift your back leg to the ceiling.

COMMON CHALLENGES Tight hips prevent you from coming down to your elbows.

MODIFICATION Place a block underneath your elbows.

SEQUENCE TRANSITION If in Bound Lizard, release your foot gently. • Come up to your hands.

Half Pigeon

BOUND VARIATION Come up to your hands. Reach your right hand for your back foot. Stay on your left hand or lower your left elbow to a block or the floor. • Slowly shift your weight toward your front foot. Stay another ten breaths. Look to a spot on the wall to the right or close your eyes. • **Modification:** If you have trouble grabbing your foot because of tightness in your hamstrings or hips, loop a strap around your foot and hold the strap for the stretch.

How do hips get tight? Let me count the ways: hiking, running, sitting, and countless more. Your muscular hips need to be both strong and flexible to climb at your most optimal, and they need extra time to relax and release. Your body may resist this stretch initially as you work into your piriformis, a deep hip stabilizer. Breathe deeply into the sensation in your body, and give the muscles around your hip time to soften as you work into the stretch.

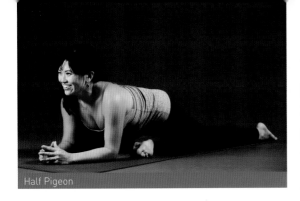
Half Pigeon

SETUP From Lizard, move your right foot across your mat and in toward your pelvis, keeping your right foot flexed to protect your knee. Extend your left leg straight behind you so that the top of your thigh is on the ground.

ALIGNMENT Flex the toes on your back foot and come up to the ball of your foot. • Roll up to center so your pelvis is squared toward the front of your mat. Place a block under your right hip if you have trouble staying centered. • Pull your thigh bones in toward your pelvis. • Lengthen your chest and slowly lower your torso toward the floor. • Walk your arms in front of you. Soften your shoulders and face.

• Place a block under your forehead if it doesn't touch your mat. • Stay for one minute.

GAZE & FOCUS Close your eyes. • Breathe deeply into your hips.

DEEPEN Shift your front shin closer to parallel with the front of your mat to get a deeper opening.

COMMON CHALLENGES Knee injuries prevent you from staying in this pose without sharp pain or you are experiencing lower back and leg pain from sciatica.

MODIFICATION Take Reclined Pigeon (see Strength Practice I for more details).

Double Pigeon

If you thought Half Pigeon was a delight, Double Pigeon will transport you into a whole new realm of hip opening. This pose is the very essence of patience! See if you can breathe deeply and relax the intensity of the pose, breathing into unexplored territory in your hips.

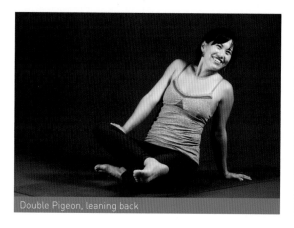
Double Pigeon, leaning back

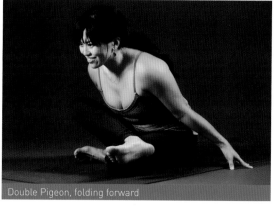
Double Pigeon, folding forward

SETUP From Half Pigeon, swing your back leg forward and around. Flex your upper foot and move it until your ankle bone is just past your thigh.
• Flex the toes of your right foot and tuck your foot in toward your pelvis.

ALIGNMENT Move around until you can ground your sit bones on the floor. • Bring your thighs parallel with the long edges of your mat. Flex both of your feet to protect your knees. • Place your left hand on your left inner thigh. Bring your right hand to the floor behind you. Press your left thigh open toward the floor. • Place your hands on either side of your hips and slowly reach your chest forward toward your legs. If you can walk your hands forward and relax, do that. • Stay for one minute.

GAZE & FOCUS Close your eyes or look at the ground in front of you. • Pay attention to the sensation in your hips and send your breath there.

DEEPEN If you have open hips, bring your lower shin in line with your upper shin. Keep your toes flexed. Lower your chest forward over your legs.

COMMON CHALLENGES Tight hips prevent you from bringing both of your sit bones to the ground.

MODIFICATION Sit on a block to take the work out of your hip flexors and into the bigger muscles around your pelvis.

SEQUENCE TRANSITION Swing your upper leg to the back of your mat. • Step your front foot toward the back edge of your mat for Downward-Facing Dog. • Step your left foot forward for Lizard through Double Pigeon on your left side. • From Downward-Facing Dog, move into a seated position.

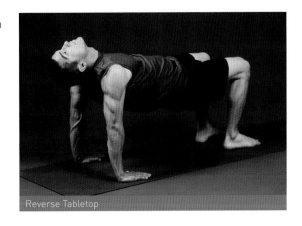
Reverse Tabletop

Reverse Tabletop

A shoulder opener, Reverse Tabletop is also a back-bend that moves deeply into your chest, biceps, and deltoids in your shoulders, an area that can use some opening after climbing. Always an interesting challenge, it's a powerful, modified backbend.

SETUP From a seated position, place your hands behind you on the mat with your fingertips facing your body. Walk your feet in so they are flat on the floor at hip-width distance.

ALIGNMENT Ground into the four corners of your feet and lift your hips toward the ceiling. • Press your palms into the ground. • Lengthen the crown of your head behind you. Gently release your head onto your shoulders. • Rotate your inner thighs toward each other and down toward your mat.

GAZE & FOCUS Set your gaze on the ceiling or wall behind you. • Ground your feet deeper into the floor to activate your leg muscles.

DEEPEN Extend your legs straight on the floor. Press into your heels to lift your hips. Press the soles of your feet into the earth; spin your inner thighs down toward the floor.

COMMON CHALLENGES Weak hamstrings make it difficult to keep your legs internally rotated. Also, tight chest muscles can make breathing feel challenging.

MODIFICATION Play with moving your breath around to stay in the pose.

SEQUENCE TRANSITION Lower your hips to the floor from Reverse Tabletop into a seated position.

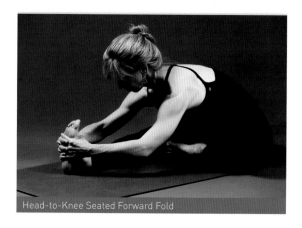
Head-to-Knee Seated Forward Fold

Head-to-Knee Seated Forward Fold

When your body is tired from practice, it is easier to relax into stretches. Use your breath to soften your muscles and get deeper into your body.

SETUP From a seated position, extend one leg straight. Tuck your other foot in toward your pelvis, bringing the sole in against your inner thigh.

ALIGNMENT Flex the toes on your extended leg.
• Reach your hands for your extended foot.
• Squeeze your thigh muscles to extend into your hamstring. • Lengthen your chest toward your foot. Release your head toward your shin. • Keep your sit bones grounded. • Hold for ten breaths.

GAZE & FOCUS Close your eyes. • Ground your sit bones into the mat.

DEEPEN On your inhale lengthen your chest toward your foot; exhale and fold deeper.

COMMON CHALLENGES Knee injuries prevent you from bringing your foot in toward your pelvis.

MODIFICATION If you can't reach your foot, use a strap or a towel. • Bring your bent foot into your shin instead of to your inner thigh.

SEQUENCE TRANSITION Repeat pose on other side. • Come to a seated position and roll down onto your back.

Shoulder Stand

Going upside down is a hallmark of a yoga practice, inverting both your body and your perspective on the world. The queen of all inversions, Shoulder Stand creates harmony in your nervous and endocrine systems. It is a restorative inversion, stimulating the heart and flushing your spine.

SETUP From your back, lift your feet up and over behind your head, reaching them toward the floor behind you so your pelvis stacks over your shoulders. Wiggle your shoulders underneath you to create a solid base. • Place your palms on your back.

ALIGNMENT Inch your shoulders in closer toward your spine to create a solid foundation. • Lift your hips and legs higher with your hands on your back by walking your elbows in toward each other. • Extend your legs up toward the ceiling. • Keep a gap between your chin and chest to keep your neck off the floor.

GAZE & FOCUS Set your drishti on the ceiling and keep it focused there; avoid turning your head from side to side—this will protect your neck. • Keep your legs still.

DEEPEN Lift your hips higher over your shoulders.

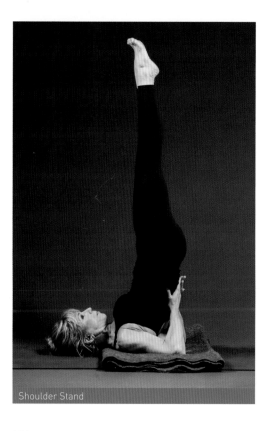
Shoulder Stand

COMMON CHALLENGES A tight lower back and/or hamstrings make it difficult to get into the pose.

MODIFICATION Place a folded blanket under your shoulders for padding before moving into the pose. Or substitute with Legs Up the Wall pose (from Strength Practice I.)

Ear Pressure Pose

Allow yourself to relax into the Ear Pressure Pose and feel the benefits of this deep stretch into the mid-back and turning your body upside-down.

SETUP From Shoulder Stand, lower your knees toward your forehead. Keep your hips stacked over your shoulders.

ALIGNMENT Keep your hands on your back; relax your mid-back. • Rest your knees on your forehead. • If your body allows, bring your knees outside your ears. • If your knees come down by your ears, wrap your arms around the backs of your thighs. Otherwise, keep your hands on your back.

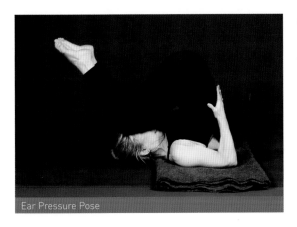
Ear Pressure Pose

GAZE & FOCUS Close your eyes. • Soften your spine and mid-back.

COMMON CHALLENGES Your back doesn't allow your knees to reach your ears.

MODIFICATION Keep your knees on your forehead.

SEQUENCE TRANSITION Roll slowly out of Ear Pressure pose. • Come up to a seated position.

A backbend counter pose to Shoulder Stand, Fish opens your chest and throat wide to the sky. Now is a perfect time to take a Lion's Breath, a big, open-mouthed *loud* exhale. Stick your tongue out to release your jaw!

SETUP From a seated position with your legs straight on the mat, slide your fingertips underneath your sit bones. Lower to your elbows, keeping your shoulders off the floor. Press into your hands and puff your chest up to the ceiling. • Lower the top of your head to the mat.

ALIGNMENT Tuck your chin to lengthen the top of your head behind you and lower your head toward the floor. • Press deeply into your hands and slide them underneath you to bring your head onto the floor. • Open your chest to the sky. • Take a Lion's Breath: Inhale deeply. On your exhale, stick out your tongue and roar loudly.

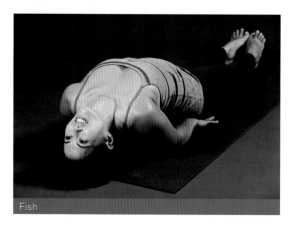

Fish

Tuck your chin to release to the floor.

Supine Twist

A Supine Twist relaxes your spine and allows your body to wind down from the intensity of practice and also to loosen your spine from the impact of gravity. (Note: Photo shows deeper option.)

SETUP From a resting position on your back, pull your knees into your chest. Extend your arms open into a T.

GAZE & FOCUS Close your eyes or look at a spot on the floor behind you. • Connect the top of your head to the floor to relax your neck. Breathe into your chest.

COMMON CHALLENGES You can't get your head to the floor.

MODIFICATION Slide your hands deeper underneath you. Or, place a block (in its widest direction) just below your shoulder blades. Relax over your block for a more restorative Fish.

ALIGNMENT Lower your knees to your left, knees still hugging in toward your chest. • Shift your hips under you toward the right. • Keep both shoulders anchored on the floor. • Look away from the twist to your right hand so your neck also benefits from the rotation. • Stay for ten breaths.

GAZE & FOCUS Look away from your knees toward your opposite hand. • Relax your body and allow

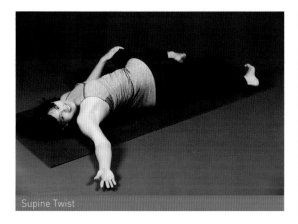

Supine Twist

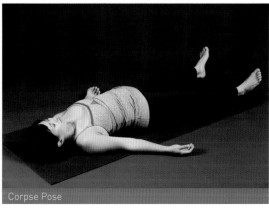

Corpse Pose

gravity to take the weight of your legs toward the floor.

DEEPEN Pull your right knee into your chest, and straighten your left leg on the ground to deepen the twist. Roll your right knee toward your left side.

SEQUENCE TRANSITION Repeat the twist on the other side of your body.

FINAL REST

You've got this one! Lay down, relax all the muscles in your body, let go of your ujjayi breath, and know that all is well.

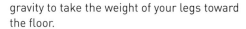

Corpse Pose

Relax all the muscles in your body, starting with your legs, moving through your hips, belly, shoulders, and face. Commit to staying still.

SETUP From Supine Twist, come to Corpse Pose with your arms at your sides, palms facing up.

ALIGNMENT Slide your shoulders under you. • Relax the muscles in your legs, shoulders, and face. • Move into your natural breath. • Stay in this pose for three minutes.

GAZE & FOCUS Close your eyes. • Stay awake and still. Notice your natural breath.

DEEPEN Take a five-minute final rest.

RECOVERY PRACTICE

TIME: 30 MINUTES
EQUIPMENT: BLOCK, YOGA MAT, STRAP, AND BOLSTER (OPTIONAL)

Pushing limits comes naturally to climbers. The sport requires focus and persistence to master the next level of climb. As a climber, you know what it's like to chase a route, taxing your body over and over again for hours at a time, and testing your physical endurance and mental strength.

Your body also is meant to rest and recover. You may be excellent at the school of recovering prone on the couch. Some days, I include myself in this category. I love a good day of doing nothing, despite the advice of my own trainers to do something every day, even on a rest day. Others of you may itch to move, unwilling to spend a day without expending any energy.

A middle ground exists between relentless action and zero. When tired, and especially when sore, you may be tempted to take the couch approach. You reason that you already spent hours outdoors, and your legs are throbbing, your shoulders ache, and your hands are fried. And the idea of movement sounds torturous, and the temptation to stay still is strong. But it is still wise to move your body—and you will move through the soreness faster by moving again.

A restorative yoga practice offers your body a soft approach, giving it the space it needs to heal from the previous day's intensity while still moving the lactic acid through your muscles to support a faster recovery.

The following practice is intended for a day you can tell you need to take it down a notch. It

SEQUENCE FOR RECOVERY PRACTICE

- » Child's Pose
- » Cat–Cow
- » Downward-Facing Dog
- » Rag Doll
- » Modified Sun Salutation A
- » Low Lunge
- » Twisted Crescent Lunge, Modified
- » Lizard
- » Squat
- » Gorilla Variation
- » Eagle
- » One-Armed Shoulder Opener
- » Locust
- » Heart Throat Nose Pose
- » Toes Pose
- » Half Pigeon
- » Double Pigeon
- » Frog
- » Reverse Tabletop
- » Head-to-Knee Seated Forward Fold with a Twist
- » Seated Twist
- » Legs Up the Wall
- » Corpse Pose

addresses the major parts of the body that need a gentler touch after an extended day climbing, including long stretches into your hips and shoulders and mellow twists to open your spine. With a focus on breathing, you will notice the sensations of your body and more easily relieve any stress you may feel.

With a 30-minute restorative yoga practice, you can hone in on areas that ache or feel like they need some attention, allowing you more time in longer stretches to release more deeply and recover with ease.

INTEGRATE AND ACTIVATE

Even in a recovery sequence, it's still important to warm the body before moving into deep stretches. Use this time to settle your mind, get connected with your body and prepare to release mentally and physically.

Child's Pose

Start your recovery practice with Child's Pose to notice your physical body and your ujjayi breath, and to bring your mind to the present. Observe

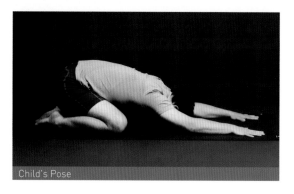
Child's Pose

in toward your spine. • Come into your ujjayi breath. • Stay for ten breaths.

GAZE & FOCUS Close your eyes. • Deepen your ujjayi breath. Pay attention to the feeling of the mat under your hands and forehead.

COMMON CHALLENGES A tight lower back or hips can prevent your forehead from touching the ground. • Knee injuries can prevent you from bending your knees comfortably.

MODIFICATIONS Bring a block under your forehead to relax your neck. • Roll over onto your back for Supine Butterfly or lay flat on your belly.

SEQUENCE TRANSITION Move forward to your hands and your knees.

the feeling of your mat underneath your hands and forehead. Feel your breath move into your ribs. Listen to what your body is telling you.

SETUP From a seat, move your knees to the edges of your mat, and bring your big toes together to touch. Sink your hips back over your heels. Walk your hands forward at shoulder-width distance and bring your forehead to the ground.

ALIGNMENT Let go of tension in your shoulders. • Engage your core gently, pulling your belly up and

Cat–Cow

Cat–Cow is a gentle way to warm up your spine, releasing tension there, including your neck. The pose creates fluidity in your pelvis and lower back,

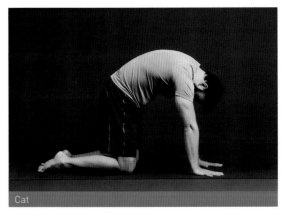

Cat

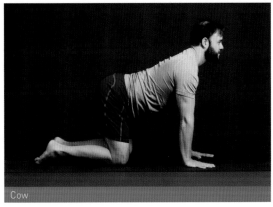

Cow

particularly if you are feeling stiff after a long day hauling gear and climbing. It also syncs your breath with your body's movement for a vinyasa flow.

SETUP On your hands and knees, stack your hands underneath your shoulders, palms flat. Stack your knees under your hips.

ALIGNMENT Pull your navel up and in toward your spine. Keep your spine neutral to start. • **Cat:** On an exhale, arch your spine and roll your shoulders forward. Keep your belly engaged as you round your spine. Move your gaze down toward your legs. • **Cow:** On an inhale, lift your tailbone and chest toward the ceiling. Soften your belly toward the floor while keeping your core engaged. Stretch the crown of your head toward the ceiling. • Repeat the Cat–Cow cycle five times.

GAZE & FOCUS Let your drishti move naturally with the pose, or work with your eyes closed. • Move your spine slowly, and let the pace of your breath determine how long it takes to do each Cat and Cow. Take your time and breathe fully.

DEEPEN Shift your hips in broad circular movements. Start clockwise, moving your right hip out past your mat, swing it back down over your heels, move to the left edge of your mat, and move your weight forward into your hands to complete a circle. Do it three times, then repeat counterclockwise three times.

SEQUENCE TRANSITION Tuck your toes and lift your hips to the ceiling for Downward-Facing Dog.

Downward-Facing Dog

As you become familiar with it, Downward-Facing Dog may evolve into the resting pose it is meant to be. Use the time in this pose to listen to your body, open into your shoulders, spine and hamstrings, and focus your gaze.

SETUP Lift your hips to the sky. Move your feet back about six inches toward the back edge of your mat.

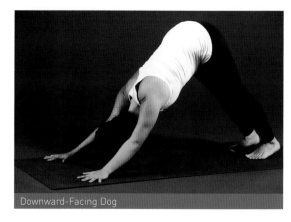
Downward-Facing Dog

ALIGNMENT Point your index fingers to the front of your mat. • Flatten your palms until the knuckles at the base of your index and middle fingers are grounded on your mat. • Move your feet to hip-width distance. Spin your inner ankles back so the outer edges of your feet are parallel with the edge of your mat. • Bend your knees and lift your tailbone toward the ceiling until your spine lengthens. • Spin your sit bones to the wall behind you. • Roll your shoulders up to your ears, then use your back muscles to pull your shoulders down your back and in toward your spine. Squeeze your upper arms toward each other. • Press your chest toward your thighs; keep your shoulders engaged and do not hyperextend in your shoulders. • Drive your heels toward the floor (they don't need to touch the floor). • Pull your belly in toward your spine. • Lift the muscles just above your knees to engage your thighs and open into your hamstrings. • Create a long line from your wrists to your shoulders and hips; bend your knees as you need to. • Stay for ten breaths.

GAZE & FOCUS Look backward at the floor between your big toes. • Lift your tailbone high toward the ceiling.

DEEPEN Once the pose feels more comfortable, press your heels deeply toward the mat until your toes can spread and soften.

COMMON CHALLENGES Tight hamstrings can lead to a rounded spine. • If you have a wrist injury, it may be painful to stay on your hands.

MODIFICATIONS For tight hamstrings, bend your knees and lift your tailbone toward the ceiling. Pull

your shoulders toward your spine. Press your chest toward your legs. • For wrist pain, come down to your elbows for Dolphin pose: Move your elbows in so they are stacked directly under your shoulders. Walk your feet in toward your elbows as close as you can. Lift your tailbone to the sky.

SEQUENCE TRANSITION Walk your feet to the front of your mat.

Rag Doll

Connect to your feet, relax your spine, and let go in your neck.

SETUP Stand with your feet hip-width distance apart. Stretch out your toes and activate your feet. Fold your chest toward the floor. Hold your elbows and hang your upper body, letting go of your head.

ALIGNMENT Lift and spread out your toes, creating gaps between every toe from your big toe to your pinky toe. • Soften your toes to the floor. Press the four corners of your feet—your big toe and pinky toe knuckles, and the two sides of your heels—into the

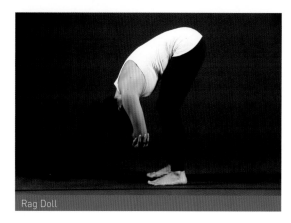
Rag Doll

floor. • Spin your inner ankles toward the back of your mat and energetically draw your outer ankles toward the floor. Notice how this lifts the arches of your feet. • Bend your knees slightly until your belly comes down to the tops of your thighs. • Squeeze your inner thighs up toward your pelvis. • Turn your head side to side to soften your neck. Stick out your tongue to release your jaw. • Sway gently side to side. • Stay for five breaths.

Close your eyes or set your gaze on a spot between your feet. • Release your spine and neck.

DEEPEN As you get more open in your hamstrings and lower back, your legs straighten more. Keep your knee joints soft in the pose.

SEQUENCE TRANSITION Release your elbows and bring your feet together.

Sun Salutation A

Follow the sequence for Sun Salutation A as outlined in Strength Practice I to warm up your body and to focus on your breath. Do three rounds.

Mountain Pose, inhale with arms up. • Forward Fold, exhale. • Halfway Lift, inhale. • Plank to floor, exhale. • Low Cobra, inhale. • Downward-Facing Dog, exhale, hold pose for five breaths. • Step or jump forward to the front of your mat. • Halfway Lift, inhale. • Forward Fold, exhale. • Mountain Pose, arms up, inhale. • Repeat sequence two more times.

Low Lunge

Focus on pulling your thigh bones in toward your pelvis to feel your center line and stretch into your hip flexors.

SETUP Move through Sun Salutation A to Downward-Facing Dog. From Downward-Facing Dog, step your right foot between your hands. Lower your back knee to the floor and point your back toes. Bring your hands to your front thigh.

ALIGNMENT Square your hips toward the front of your mat. Pull your front foot and back knee toward each other to integrate. Your hips will lift slightly higher than before. • Once your centerline is established, slowly shift your weight forward toward your front foot. Stack your front knee over your ankle. • Squeeze your belly in toward your spine and hug your front ribs together. • Reach your arms up toward the ceiling, palms facing in. Breathe deeply into the stretch in your hip flexor. • Stay for five breaths.

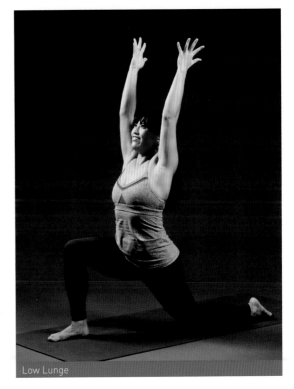

Low Lunge

GAZE & FOCUS Look at a spot on the wall in front of you. • Hug your thigh bones in toward each other to keep your body strong while opening into your hip.

DEEPEN Tuck your back toes and lift your heel vertically over the ball of your foot for Crescent Lunge (see Strength Practice II).

COMMON CHALLENGES Your knee hurts on the ground.

MODIFICATION Fold over an edge of your mat to pad your knee.

Twisted Crescent Lunge

Move gently into a twist to activate your core and back muscles and release your spine from a vigorous day climbing. Keep your back knee on the floor to take the intensity down.

SETUP From Low Lunge, place your right hand to the inside of your front foot on a block or the floor. • Extend your left hand in line with your shoulder. On an inhale, stretch your chest longer to get more

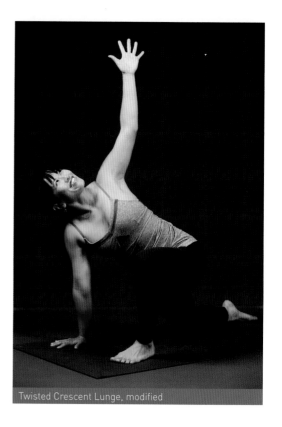

Twisted Crescent Lunge, modified

space in your spine. On an exhale, move deeper into the twist in your mid-back.

ALIGNMENT Shift your weight forward toward your left foot, keeping your knee pointing forward over your ankle; don't let it cave in or out. • Lengthen your spine through the crown of your head to create more space for the twist. • Pull your shoulder blades toward your spine, and engage the muscles under your shoulder blades to deepen your twist. • Pull your belly in toward your spine. • Stretch your upper fingers out wide and toward the ceiling. • Stay for five breaths.

GAZE & FOCUS Set your gaze on a spot on the ceiling. • Squeeze your shoulder blades toward each other. Spin your chest toward the ceiling.

MODIFICATION Pad your knee if you feel pain in your kneecap.

SEQUENCE TRANSITION Bring your hands to the floor on either side of your front foot to a Low Lunge.

Lizard

Your body may resist the intensity of this hip-opening pose at first. Use your breath to release deep into your hips.

SETUP From Low Lunge, bring both hands to the floor inside your front leg. Angle your toes on your front foot to the outer edge of your mat.

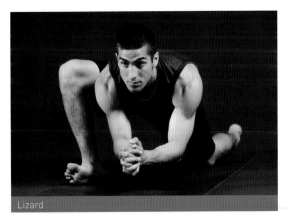

Lizard

ALIGNMENT Flex your front foot and roll to the outer edge of your foot. The sole of your foot is off the floor and your right knee will roll open. • Lower your elbows down beside your foot with elbows roughly in line with your heel. • Release your head toward your hands. • Stay for ten breaths.

GAZE & FOCUS Look at the inside of your front foot. • Notice the sensations in your hip and send your breath there.

BOUND LIZARD VARIATION While still in Lizard, come up to your hands. Reach your right hand for your back foot. Stay on your left hand or lower your left elbow to a block or the floor. Slowly shift your weight toward your front foot. Stay another ten breaths. Look to a spot on the wall to the right, or close your eyes. If you have trouble grabbing your foot because of tightness in your hamstrings or hips, loop a strap around your foot and hold the strap for the stretch.

DEEPEN Do not bind your Lizard. Instead, tuck your back toes, squeeze your quads, and lift your back leg to the ceiling.

COMMON CHALLENGES Tight hips prevent you from coming down to your elbows.

MODIFICATION Place a block underneath your elbows. • Let go of your back foot gently.

SEQUENCE TRANSITION If in Bound Lizard, release your foot gently. • Come back up to your hands. Bring your right foot flat and pointed forward to the front of your mat. • Press your hands into the mat and step back to Downward-Facing Dog. • Do Low Lunge through Lizard on your left side. • Move to Downward-Facing Dog. • Step to the top of your mat.

Squat

Allow yourself to settle into a squat, opening into your spine and your hips. Breathe in deeply and let your hips sink a little more toward the floor.

SETUP Walk your feet as wide as your mat. Bend your knees to lower your hips toward the floor. If your heels lift off the floor, widen your stance until you can get your feet flat. Your toes can turn out wider than your heels. • Bring your hands together, palms touching, in front of your chest.

ALIGNMENT Shift your weight into the outer arches of your feet, and lift your inner arches. Squeeze your heels in toward each other like you are trying to wrinkle your mat. • Lift your belly button in toward your spine to lift your chest toward the ceiling. • Press your elbows into your inner knees. • Stay for ten breaths.

GAZE & FOCUS Set your gaze on a spot on the wall ahead. • Lengthen your spine and keep your knees aligned over your feet. Play with sitting in a passive squat, then engage your pelvic floor and lift your hips an inch out of the bottom of the squat into an active one.

DEEPEN Bring your feet wider and lower your tail-bone closer toward the floor. Work your feet toward parallel.

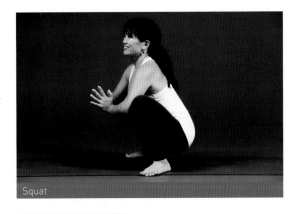
Squat

COMMON CHALLENGES Tight hips prevent you from grounding your heels.

MODIFICATION If you have trouble lowering down below your knees, stay in a higher squat position or bring a folded blanket under your heels.

SEQUENCE TRANSITION From a Squat, fold your chest forward over your legs.

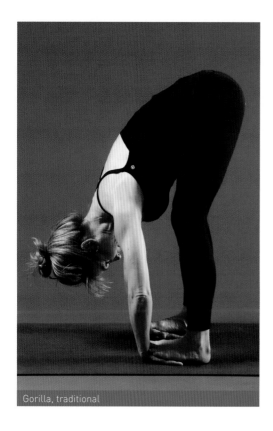

Gorilla, traditional

Gorilla Variation

It's wise to spend some time releasing your forearms and wrists after climbing. Be forewarned this variation on Gorilla takes the intensity of release to another level, particularly for tight climber hands and wrists. Be gentle and keep breathing through the pose.

SETUP Measure two fists between your feet for hip-width distance. Lift the arches of your feet and bend your knees. Turn your fingers to face in toward your feet, palms facing down and thumbs spinning out.
• Slide your hands underneath your feet like you do in a traditional Gorilla. Bend your elbows to pull your chest down toward your feet. Shift your weight slowly toward your wrists to open more deeply into your wrists and forearms. • Stay for ten breaths.

ALIGNMENT Wiggle your hands deeper under your feet until your toes reach your wrists. • Bend your elbows, and pull your shoulder blades together.
• Pull your chest deeper toward your spine. • Soften

your knees and bring your belly down to your thighs. Engage your thigh muscles. • Release your neck and hang your head toward the floor.

GAZE & FOCUS Look at the floor behind your feet. • Engage your shoulders and back muscles to pull your chest closer to your shins.

DEEPEN Work your legs as straight as your hamstrings allow while still squeezing your thighs. Keep your knee joints soft.

COMMON CHALLENGES Tight hamstrings prevent you from sliding your hands under your feet.

MODIFICATION Place your hands in the same position (fingers facing your feet, thumbs facing out) in front of your feet, or place them in that position on a block. Bend your knees.

SEQUENCE TRANSITION Release your hands from under your feet. • Bring your feet together. • Stand in Mountain Pose.

Eagle

If you're not feeling like an old pro at the Eagle bind for your arms just yet, focus on your standing foot, core, and gaze. The shoulder opening will come with time.

SETUP From Mountain Pose, extend your arms out wide and parallel to the floor, palms facing forward. Cross your right upper arm underneath your left upper arm. Wind your forearms around each other. Bring your palms to touch for the full bind. • Lower into Chair in your legs. Cross your right thigh on top of your left thigh.

ALIGNMENT Ground into your standing foot. Squeeze your inner thighs all the way together. • Stretch out your toes on your upper foot. • Stack your shoulders over your hips; engage your core lock. • Lift your elbows level with your shoulders. Press your hands away from your face to stack your wrists over your elbows. • Soften your shoulders away from your ears; pull your arm bones in toward your shoulder sockets. • Stay for five breaths.

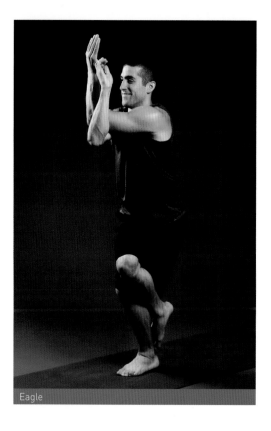
Eagle

GAZE & FOCUS Look past your arms to a spot on the wall. • Engage your belly firmly and set your gaze.

DEEPEN Bend your standing leg deeper and wrap your right foot around your calf. Challenge yourself by moving your gaze in to your forearms.

COMMON CHALLENGES Tight shoulders can prevent you from taking a full bind.

MODIFICATION Reach for opposite shoulders and lift your elbows even with your shoulders.

SEQUENCE TRANSITION Release into Mountain Pose. • Do Eagle on your left side, wrapping your left arm under your right and lifting your left leg over your right thigh. • Inhale and reach your arms up to the ceiling to release. • Fold your chest forward to your feet and exhale. • Lengthen your chest to Halfway Lift, and inhale. • Step back to Plank. • Shift to your toes and lower to the floor.

One-Armed Shoulder Opener

Many poses you have learned strengthen your shoulders. This pose is a passive stretch deep into your shoulder girdle, reversing your body's inclination from climbing and sitting to hunch forward. It also supports the mobility of your shoulder joint and can provide release for your upper back, where many people hold stress. Don't force this pose; breathe deeply into the sensations in your shoulder.

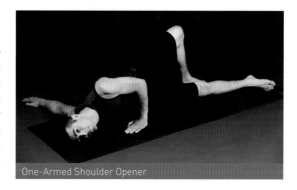

One-Armed Shoulder Opener

SETUP From your belly on the floor, extend your right arm out so your wrist is level with your eyes, palm down. Place your left hand next to your ribs on the floor, elbow bent at a 90-degree angle to the floor. • Roll over onto your right hip, bend your left leg and set your foot on the floor behind your right leg. Rest your temple on the floor or on a block.

ALIGNMENT With your left hand, which has leverage, press gently into the floor until your body naturally stops you. • Relax your shoulder and your face. • Stay for ten full breaths.

GAZE & FOCUS Look at the floor or close your eyes. • Relax into the pose. Stay focused on your breath.

DEEPEN If your body allows, bend your lower leg and place your foot flat on the floor parallel with your left foot, like a bridge. • Reach your left hand up toward the ceiling, wind it behind your body, reaching for your extended lower hand to bind. Keep your lower hand in line with your shoulder.

COMMON CHALLENGES If you have a shoulder injury, particularly in your rotator cuff, your shoulder may not allow you to do this stretch.

MODIFICATION Substitute Locust pose with a bind at your lower back. See below.

SEQUENCE TRANSITION Roll onto your belly to release. • Do One-Armed Shoulder Opener on your left side.

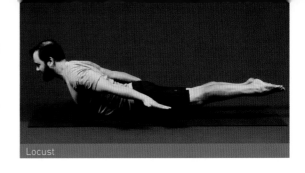
Locust

Locust

Now that you have experience with backbends, keep your legs strong and lift from your belly and chest to open your shoulders and strengthen your back.

SETUP On your belly, bring your feet to hip-width distance, toes pointed. Reach your arms alongside your body, hands down by your hips, palms facing down.

ALIGNMENT Press the tops of your feet into the floor, and lift your knees off the ground. • Keep your upper legs engaged, and lift them off the floor. • Lengthen the crown of your head forward, and lengthen and lift your chest to the ceiling. Pull your shoulders in toward your spine. • Lift your upper arm bones toward the ceiling and float your hands above your hips. • Pull your belly up and in to lift even higher into the pose. • Stay for five breaths.

BOUND VARIATION Interlace your hands at your lower back. If you have tight shoulders and cannot bind, hold a strap with your hands to modify. Lift your hands off your lower back in the pose.

GAZE & FOCUS Look past your nose at the front edge of your mat or the floor. • Squeeze your legs, engage your core, and lift from your chest forward and up to the sky.

DEEPEN Bring your inner thighs and ankles together and lift.

COMMON CHALLENGES You feel lower back strain.

MODIFICATION Keep the tops of your feet on the floor. Place your hands by your lower ribs. • Lift your chest into Low Cobra.

SEQUENCE TRANSITION Lower slowly to the floor from Locust. Wiggle your hips side to side to release your back. • Do a second Locust with the Bound Variation. • Plant your hands next to your chest and press up to your hands and knees.

Heart Throat Nose Pose

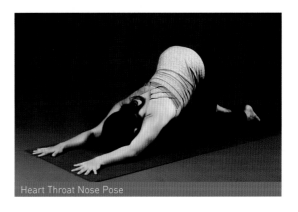

Heart Throat Nose Pose

Another shoulder and heart opener, Heart Throat Nose pose can feel comforting because we face the floor rather than the open air above. It creates a big opening into your chest and shoulders while maintaining a grounding quality.

SETUP From hands and knees, walk your arms forward, keeping your hips stacked over your knees, until your forehead comes to the ground.

ALIGNMENT Activate your core to protect your lower back. • Melt the space between your shoulders toward the floor; soften your chest toward the ground. • Stay for five breaths.

GAZE & FOCUS Set your gaze on the floor or close your eyes. • Engage your core and soften into your upper back.

DEEPEN If your shoulders are open enough so your chest touches the floor, lift your chin and place it on the floor.

Walk your hands in and come to a seated position on your knees.

Toes Pose

Your feet, ankles, and calves work intensely on holds, mastering balance points on your toes. In addition, most people spend at least some of their day up on the balls of their feet in shoes with a slightly lifted heel rather than flexing their feet and working into their Achilles tendon. Toes Pose stretches into the soles of your feet and can be an intense stretch. Breathe!

SETUP Tuck your toes underneath you until you are on the ball of your foot—tuck your pinky toe in if it escapes. Sit up slowly and lift your chest over your hips until you feel the sensation in your feet.

ALIGNMENT If the pose is immediately too intense, lean forward for a moment, then return to lift your chest upright. • Engage your core lock. • Stay for ten full breaths. • **Counter pose**: Shift forward onto hands and knees. Release your toe tuck and point your toes on the floor. Bring your hands by your hips

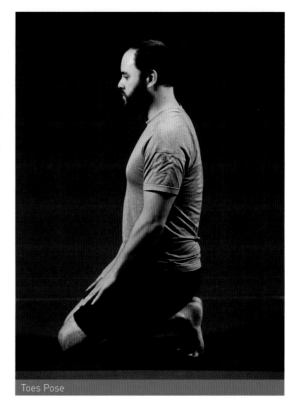

Toes Pose

and lean back to stretch into your shins, the front of your foot and your ankles in the opposite direction to counter the intensity. • Stay for ten breaths.

GAZE & FOCUS Set your gaze on a spot on the wall. • Notice if your mind wants to take you out of the pose. Stay with the pose.

DEEPEN Hold for twenty breaths.

COMMON CHALLENGES Knee pain prevents you from taking the pose.

MODIFICATIONS Roll up a blanket (or small towel) and place it behind your knees or on top of your ankles

SEQUENCE TRANSITION Move to a seated position on your sit bones and set up for Half Pigeon.

RELEASE AND RESTORE

It's time to move into poses that both release and restore your body. Your trunk and lower body have shouldered much of the work. Focus on breathing and releasing in these deep stretches.

Half Pigeon

By now, you may have a new appreciation for the release available in your hips. Challenge yourself to stay in Half Pigeon longer than you have before.

SETUP From a seated position, move your right foot across your mat and in toward your pelvis, keeping your right foot flexed to protect your knee. Extend your left leg straight behind you so that the top of your thigh is on the ground.

ALIGNMENT Flex the toes on your back foot and come up to the ball of your foot. • Roll up to center so your pelvis is squared toward the front of your mat. Place a block under your right hip if you have trouble staying centered. • Pull your thigh bones in toward your pelvis. • Lengthen your chest and slowly lower your torso toward the floor. • Walk your arms in front of you. Soften your shoulders and face. • Place a block under your forehead if it doesn't touch your mat. • Stay for one minute.

GAZE & FOCUS Close your eyes. • Breathe deeply into your hips.

ACTIVE & PASSIVE RELEASE

Your brain is in constant conversation with your muscles while you stretch so it's helpful to understand how you can release. If you're not making much progress in mobility, you may not be stretching the targeted muscles. Follow cues in the poses to stretch into the appropriate part of your body.

Passive release: When you are doing passive stretches, you use body weight, gravity, and muscles to stretch. A stretch held for a longer period of time will also stretch into fascia, the connective tissue holding your body together. You never want to force your body into a stretch, which causes the muscles to contract and blocks the deepening of the stretch. Work slowly, breathing to release into the muscle. Holding a passive stretch for thirty to sixty seconds gives the muscle time to relax.

Active release: Here, you focus on a combination of muscles for release by contracting one muscle targeted for the stretch to let another muscle relax and deepen in. For example, your thigh muscles extend or straighten your knee. Contracting your thighs also signal the hamstrings to relax. In a Seated Forward Fold, you reach for your feet and straighten your legs to stretch your hamstrings. But if you soften slightly at the knee, then contract your thigh muscle to straighten your knee again, you signal the muscle to soften and you will get even deeper into the stretch.

In another method of stretching, sometimes called ballistic, your body remembers the length of muscles from the last time you practiced. Each time you do a Sun Salutation, your muscles reset to the length from the last time you did yoga. Essentially, you are opening muscles throughout your entire practice, not just when you stretch at the end.

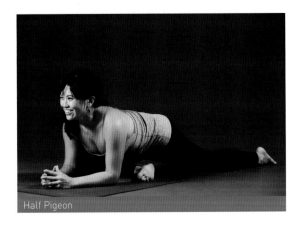
Half Pigeon

DEEPEN Shift your front shin closer to parallel with the front of your mat to get a deeper opening.

COMMON CHALLENGES Knee injuries prevent you from staying in this pose without sharp pain.

MODIFICATION Take Reclined Pigeon (see Strength Practice I for more details).

SEQUENCE TRANSITION From Half Pigeon, sweep your back leg forward to set up for Double Pigeon.

Double Pigeon

If you haven't made friends with Double Pigeon yet, the best way is more practice, of course. See if you can relax and deepen into hip opening.

SETUP From Half Pigeon, swing your back leg forward and around. Flex your upper foot and move it until your ankle is just past your thigh. Flex the toes of your lower foot and tuck it in toward your pelvis.

ALIGNMENT Move around until you can ground your sit bones on the floor. • Bring your thighs parallel with the long edges of your mat. Flex both of your feet to protect your knees. • Place your left hand on your inner thigh. Bring your right hand to the floor behind you. Press your left thigh open toward the floor. • Place your hands on either side of your hips and slowly reach your chest forward toward your legs. If you can walk your hands forward and relax, do that. • Stay for one minute.

GAZE & FOCUS Close your eyes or look at the ground in front of you. • Pay attention to the sensation in your hips and send your breath there.

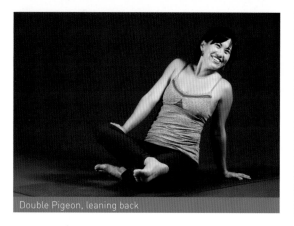

Double Pigeon, leaning back

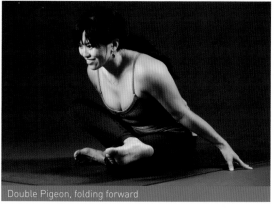

Double Pigeon, folding forward

DEEPEN If you have open hips, bring your lower shin in line with your upper shin. Keep your toes flexed. Lower your chest forward over your legs.

COMMON CHALLENGES Tight hips prevent you from bringing both of your sit bones to the ground.

MODIFICATION Sit on a block to take the work out of your hip flexors and into the bigger muscles around your pelvis.

SEQUENCE TRANSITION Unwind your legs from Double Pigeon to a seated position. • Tuck your left foot in toward your pelvis to set up for Half and Double Pigeon on the left side. • Bring both feet to the floor and sway your knees side to side to release.

Frog

An intense pose that moves into your inner thighs and groin, Frog may take some time to love. But once you fall, you fall deeply. It takes practice to stay in the pose for more than a few breaths, but it's worth pursuing: you will open deeply into new regions of your hips, and learn more about how to stay in one place when confronted with challenge, akin to the experience you have on challenging climbs.

SETUP Fold up the short edges of your mat to pad your knees. Bring your inner knees wider than hip-width distance apart on the padded edges. • Come down to your elbows (you will be off the long edge of your mat). Move your feet to a 90-degree angle with your knees. Flex your feet and bring your inner ankles to the floor. • Stack a block under your forehead.

ALIGNMENT Ensure your hips are even with your knees. • If you don't feel sensation, move your knees wider. • Pull your thigh bones in toward your pelvis. • Stay for two minutes.

GAZE & FOCUS Close your eyes. • Stay with your breath and focus on the slow release in your groin.

DEEPEN Stay longer! Try staying in this pose for up to three or four minutes, and see what happens.

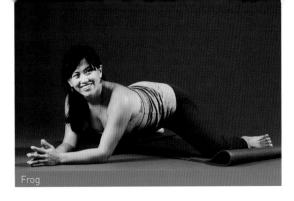
Frog

SEQUENCE TRANSITION Slowly slide forward onto your belly. • Press up to hands and knees. • Come to a seated position at the front of your mat.

Reverse Tabletop

A modified backbend that releases into your chest and shoulders, Reverse Tabletop also helps your body release from the intensity of Frog.

SETUP From a seated position, place your hands behind you on the mat with your fingertips facing your body. Walk your feet in so they are flat on the floor at hip-width distance.

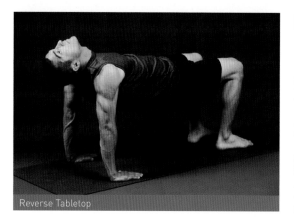
Reverse Tabletop

COMMON CHALLENGES Weak hamstrings make it difficult to keep your legs internally rotated. • Tight chest muscles can make breathing feel challenging.

MODIFICATION Play with moving your breath around to stay in the pose.

SEQUENCE TRANSITION Lower your hips to the floor.

Head-to-Knee Seated Forward Fold with a Twist

By adding a twist (not pictured), this pose works spinal length and also moves into your side body.

ALIGNMENT Ground into the four corners of your feet and lift your hips toward the ceiling. • Press your palms into the ground. • Rotate your inner thighs toward each other and down toward your mat. • Tuck your chin, lengthen the crown of your head behind you and gently release your head onto your shoulders. • Stay for five breaths.

GAZE & FOCUS Set your gaze on the ceiling or wall behind you. • Ground your feet deeper into the floor to activate your leg muscles.

SETUP From a seated position, extend your right leg toward the top right corner of your mat. Tuck your left foot in to your inner thigh. Flex your toes on your extended leg. • Twist by placing your right forearm on your right shin or lower it just inside your shin to the floor. Extend your left arm up to the ceiling. Hug your left shoulder in toward your spine.

DEEPEN Reach your upper hand toward your right foot, palm facing down. Rotate your chest toward the ceiling. If you can reach your foot, hold on to

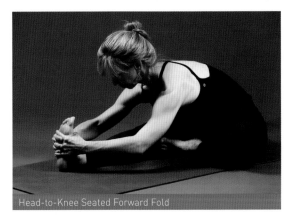

Head-to-Knee Seated Forward Fold

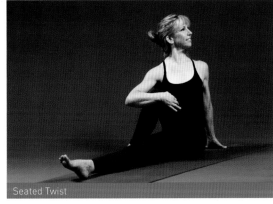

Seated Twist

your big toe. Make sure to spin your chest toward the sky. • Stay for ten rounds of breath.

SEQUENCE TRANSITION Do Head-to-Knee Seated Forward Fold with a Twist on your left side.

Seated Twist

Release your spine gently from practice through a seated twist.

SETUP Extend your right leg straight to the front of your mat, toes flexed. Place your left foot on the floor outside your right thigh. • Place your left hand on the floor behind you. Reach your right arm up to the ceiling. Wrap your right arm around your bent leg.

ALIGNMENT Lengthen your spine on your inhale. Twist toward your bent leg on your exhale. • Move your gaze past your left shoulder. • Stay for five breaths.

FOCUS Inhale to lengthen your spine and exhale to deepen your twist.

DEEPEN Hook your right elbow outside your left leg. Cross your lower leg underneath you.

SEQUENCE TRANSITION Do the Seated Twist on your right side. • Slowly roll down your back to the floor.

Legs Up the Wall

If you haven't tried this pose at the wall, this is the moment. You'll truly appreciate this restorative inversion after all of the release in this sequence.

SETUP Move your mat to a wall. Come to a seated position by the wall, and bring your left hip to touch the base of the wall. Lower yourself down to your back, and lift your legs up the wall at the same time. Scoot your sit bones to touch the wall.

ALIGNMENT Press your feet into the wall, lift your hips, and slide a block underneath your lower back. • Relax your legs. • Soften your shoulders, face, and hands. • Stay for ten breaths or longer.

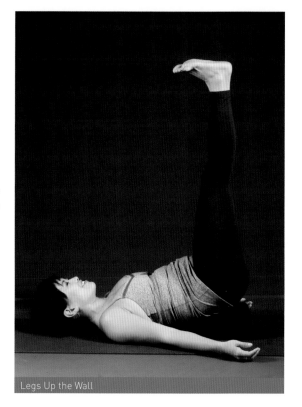
Legs Up the Wall

GAZE & FOCUS Close your eyes. • Breathe deeply and relax. Keep your legs still.

SEQUENCE TRANSITION If you are coming out of Legs Up the Wall, pull your knees to your chest and roll to one side. • Move onto your back.

FINAL REST

You can stay in Legs Up the Wall pose for your Final Rest—it's a wonderful modification that restores your body. Or, if you would like to rest in Corpse Pose, come back to the floor.

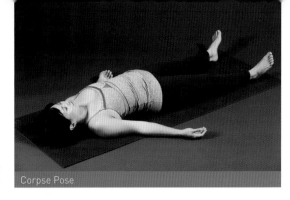

Corpse Pose

Corpse Pose

Observe how Corpse Pose feels after a slower practice.

SETUP From your back, straighten your legs on your mat. With your arms at your sides, turn your palms to face the sky.

ALIGNMENT Slide your shoulders under you.
• Relax the muscles in your legs, shoulders, and

face. • Move into your natural breath. • Close your eyes. • Stay in this pose for three minutes.

GAZE & FOCUS Close your eyes. • Stay awake and still. Notice your natural breath.

DEEPEN Take a five-minute final rest.

SUPPORTED FINAL REST Sweeten your Final Rest with a bolster. Come up to a seated position. Place a bolster lengthwise at the base of your spine. Lay down along the bolster. • Release your hands to the floor. Close your eyes. Ahh!

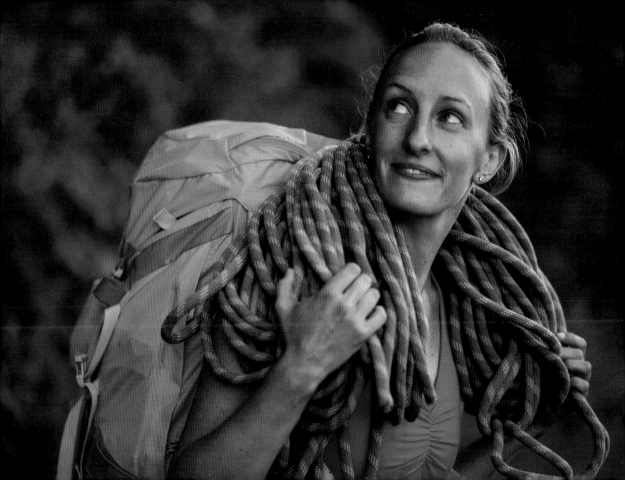

CHAPTER 5
YOGA PRACTICES FOR BEFORE AND AFTER YOU CLIMB

ANY CLIMBER ALREADY KNOWS that warm-ups are essential to a day out on the rock—maybe a few runs at an easy boulder. Or if you are out sport climbing, you probably do a few jumping jacks or traverse on the rock for a few moves to get your body ready for the long day.

Adding in a few yoga poses will add some dynamic stretches into other areas, including your hips, torso, and spine in addition to your shoulders and arms. Bring in some twists to fire up your back muscles, and you'll find it easier to turn your body for a complicated move. Plank will warm up your core, hands, and elbows, and One-Legged Chair and Low Lunge will help to access your high step faster.

A yoga practice also offers mindfulness, whether you are climbing outside or headed to the gym. Practice breathing and being present before you climb, and you will more quickly tap into that feeling of calm during the climb ahead.

At the end of your day, doing some poses to unwind will help your body recover, particularly if you are out all day on multipitch climbs or you have bouldered for hours. Do a few poses before you leave, while your body is still warm. It doesn't take much effort and the rewards are worth it.

PRE-CLIMB PRACTICE

» Stop and stand still for a moment. Look around. Note the place around you, whether it's a gym or the mountains. Observe the temperature of the space on your skin. What do you smell? What can you see? Do you see people on the rock wall or the contrast of dark mountains against blue sky? Do you hear people shouting "take" or the whistle of wind through the trees?
» Breathe deeply for five breaths.
» Find a fairly even surface. Do a few yoga poses.

Mountain Pose

» Stand with your feet together.
» Reach your arms up to the sky. Feel the great stretch in your spine.
» Lift your face to the sky. Breathe deeply for five full rounds.

Squat

» Stand with your feet wider than your shoulders.
» Lower your hips down between your feet so your hips dip below your knees.

» Press your elbows into your inner knees.
» Lift your chest up to the sky. Stay for ten breaths.

Rag Doll

» Stand with your feet at hip-width distance.
» Bend your legs slightly at the knee.
» Fold your chest forward over your legs.
» Interlace your fingers at your lower back to bind your hands.
» Stretch your arms away from your back. Stay for five breaths.

Horse Stance Twists

» Stand with your feet a leg's length distance apart from each other, turning both feet out.
» Bend your knees, tracking your knees over your ankles in the direction of your toes.
» Bring your hands to your inner thighs, and press until your arms are straight.
» Lower your right shoulder toward your left foot for a twist with your core engaged for five breaths.
» Come back to neutral. Lower your left shoulder toward your right foot for five breaths.

One-Legged Chair

» Stand with your feet together. Lower your hips toward the ground for Chair pose.
» Cross your right ankle over your left knee. Flex your upper foot.
» Insert your thumbs into your hip crease (the indentation where the top of your leg meets your hip socket), and press your hips back until you feel a stretch in your hip in your bent leg.
» Hold for five breaths. Repeat on the left side.
» Alternative: Hold onto a tree or use a boulder or a wall for balance.

Low Lunge

» Stand with your feet together. Step your left foot back and lower your left knee to the ground.
» Pull your left hip toward your right knee. Pull in your belly toward your spine.
» Lift your arms up parallel to your ears.
» Stay for five breaths.
» Bring your hands back to the ground. Step your back foot up to your right foot.
» Do the pose on the other side.

Plank

» Bring your hands to the ground. Step back to Plank Stack your hands under your shoulders. Squeeze your legs straight.
» Keep your hips just below level with your shoulders. Pull your arm bones into your shoulder sockets, squeezing them toward each other, and stretch your chest long.
» Stay for twenty rounds of breath.

POST-CLIMB PRACTICE

Climbing is intense, and these poses will help your body ease out of your time on the wall. Add the following poses after you complete the Pre-Climb Practice (above) sequence to help release your hips and lower back. Take off your climbing shoes and stretch out your toes! Do all the poses in order on your right side, then switch to your left.

Twisted Crescent Lunge, Modified

» From Mountain pose, step your left foot behind you to a Low Lunge with your right foot in front, and your back knee on the ground behind you.

» Lower your left hand to the ground; squeeze your inner thighs in toward your pelvis.
» Stretch your right fingers up to the sky. Hug your shoulder blades toward your spine.
» Engage your core lock. Look up past your right hand to the clouds. Stay for five breaths.

Triangle

» From your Low Lunge, tuck your back toes and spin your back heel toe the ground. Stack your front knee over your ankle, and lift your chest over your hips for Warrior 2.
» Keeping your front foot facing forward, straighten your front leg.
» Reach your front hand forward until your right ribs are parallel to the ground.
» Lower your right hand to your right shin. Stretch your left fingers to the sky and look up past your left hand.
» Stay for five breaths.

Skandasana

» Come up to stand from Triangle.
» Spin your right foot parallel with your left foot.
» Turn your left toes out slightly at an angle, and bend your left knee over your left ankle.
» Keep your right leg straight. Bring your hands to the ground under your shoulders.
» Lift your chest even with your hips. Stick your sit bones out behind you.
» Pull your belly in toward your back.
» Stay for five breaths.

Lizard

» Shift your weight forward into a Low Lunge. Bring your hands to the ground inside your right foot.
» Turn your right toes out at an angle, and roll to the outer edge of your foot. Keep your foot flexed.
» Stay here with hands on the ground or deepen by bringing your forearms to the ground.
» Stay for five breaths.

Half Pigeon

» Come up to your hands from Lizard.
» Walk your right foot in front of your body until your right knee comes to the ground. Keep your foot flexed.
» Square your hips toward the ground. Lift your chest up and lengthen your spine.
» Slowly lower your chest to the ground.
» If you have knee pain, modify with a Reclined Half Pigeon on your back from Strength Practice I.
» Stay for ten breaths.
» Sequence Transition: Complete Twisted Crescent Lunge through Half Pigeon on the right side, then do the poses on your left side. Move to a seat for Toes Pose.

Toes Pose

» If you haven't yet, take your shoes off for this closing pose.
» Come to your knees on the ground.
» Tuck your toes underneath you until you are on the balls of your feet—tuck your pinky toes in if they escape.
» Slowly sit back on your feet to stretch the soles of your feet and your Achilles tendon.
» Stay for ten breaths.
» Counter pose: Shift forward onto your hands and knees. Release your toe tuck and point your toes on the floor. Bring your hands to the ground behind you and lean back on your feet to stretch into your shins, the front of your foot and your ankles in the opposite direction to counter the intensity.

Wall Shoulder Stretch

» Modify a floor shoulder-opening pose by doing this against a rock wall.
» Face the wall, standing up straight with your chest touching the wall.
» Extend your right arm out 90 degrees so your fingers are just above shoulder height.
» Slowly spin your body to the right until you feel an opening in your right shoulder. Keep your body flush to the wall.
» Stay for ten breaths.
» Switch sides.

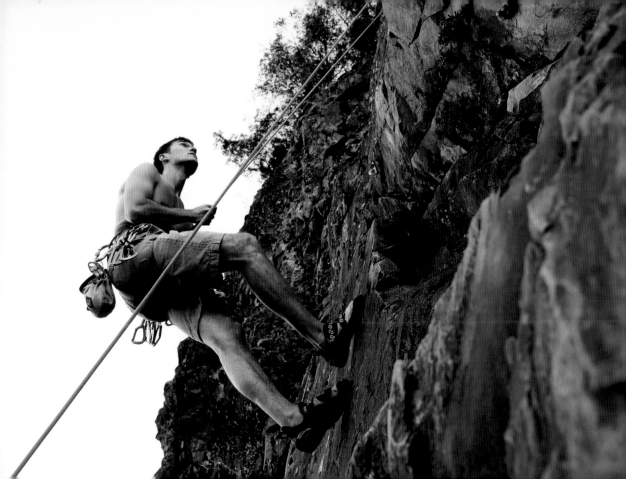

CHAPTER 6
FINDING A YOGA CLASS

I WAS MINDING MY own practice in class. My sister was with me; we were there to move, breathe, and get a break from the family vacation we were on in Taiwan. I was content to be in a challenging yoga class under the watchful eye of Patrick Creelman, an experienced teacher for the Pure Yoga franchise in Asia.

The class was up in Wheel pose. Patrick came over to me as I was getting ready to take my Wheel. "Move your feet closer together," he said. I felt a twinge of annoyance. I knew his instructions would make the pose harder. He used his feet to inch mine closer together. I went up. Yep, harder. I also felt the backbend go deeper. My legs were shaking from the intensity.

We came down, and he called for another. Out of habit or rebelliousness, I can't say for sure, I inched my feet out wider. He came back to me and said, "Bring your feet closer together." I got the message. *You're strong enough. You can do this.*

You can learn many things in a home yoga practice; with breath, a focus on your feet and alignment, and a quiet space, you can move through a deeper understanding of your body, and shift your energy and mental space. It's the same energy you feel when you are focused on a climb, easily making moves you have struggled with before. You focus, you breathe, and you move upward.

But at some point, everyone needs to get *checked*, as Patrick told the class that day. A teacher is like the hardcore friend who tells you that you're capable of doing the next level of climb, or doesn't tell you what the level is to begin with. You don't think, you just go.

When I encounter a yoga teacher like Patrick, I remember why it's so important to be held accountable. If I practice alone, I can't always see the next step in my practice. Or, even if I do see it, I talk myself out of doing it. Without anyone there to keep an eye on me, I might give up on myself. Practicing with a great teacher is a way of giving back to yourself. You will learn new poses, see new possibilities in your practice, and become immersed in a new community—another impactful reason to take a class.

I have practiced with hundreds of people at trainings. The words of my teachers landed in my body and chest, and opened me up in ways I had never felt before, physically and energetically. I remember feeling at times in final rest a deep sense of freedom; contentment; and true, uplifted joy akin to being outside challenging my body on a cool, perfect day with the people I love most in the world.

A guided practice also offers a different kind of freedom: You don't have to think about the next pose or where to move your feet or hands. A teacher leads the way.

As you take on these practices and get stronger, the next step will be finding a place to elevate your practice. While it is useful to understand the basics of the types of yoga available, it is more important to find a place that fits with your overall intention for your practice. With so many options available, the search can feel challenging. Start with the easy options, such as a nearby community center, your office, or the classes at your gym. If none of those feel quite right, take advantage of a yoga studio's introductory offer, lasting from one week to one month, giving you a chance to take classes from multiple instructors and see if the studio community is a fit.

If one doesn't work out, try another. It's important to find the one that suits you. Follow the four steps below to define what you want to get from a yoga class. *Stay open to the process!*

STEP 1: CHOOSE AN ENVIRONMENT

Identify what kind of environment you want to practice in. For some people, the convenience of a workplace class trumps practicing in a conference room! For others, classes at the gym work well. For those of you looking for a deeper quiet with like-minded people, a yoga studio may be the best fit. No matter where you go, try more than one teacher at a location, particularly if the place offers different styles.

WORKPLACE

Some workplaces now offer their employees yoga classes. These classes are frequently subsidized and so may be offered at a lower drop-in rate than they would be at a yoga studio. You will also get to know your coworkers in a different space. I taught a corporate class where the CEO showed up every week. You never know who will be practicing next to you!

GYM

Most classes are included in your gym membership, so it's a convenient, low-cost way to experience a guided class with a teacher who can check your form. Many climbing gyms are now offering regular yoga classes. Drawbacks may include a louder environment than you'd like, with people coming and going during the session. Take advantage of a class after an evening climb.

YOGA STUDIOS

Yoga studios offer more daily classes and likely more variety in style than the gym or your workplace, although some specialize. The environment is designed to be clear and calming with an intention to create community. The best yoga studios foster powerful communities where teachers and students know one another, connect on a personal level, and are part of each other's daily lives. If you are looking to deepen your practice, a studio also generally offers workshops and trainings to give you more guidance.

STEP 2: IDENTIFY A STYLE THAT SPEAKS TO YOU

As yoga has exploded in popularity in the United States, the number of styles continues to expand. From a gentle yin practice to relax your body to flow practices where people pop upside down into handstands at every opportunity, the choices are vast. The following guidelines are broad, but will get you started. The following styles are listed roughly in order from more vigorous practices to more gentle, though that may vary depending on your idea of challenge!

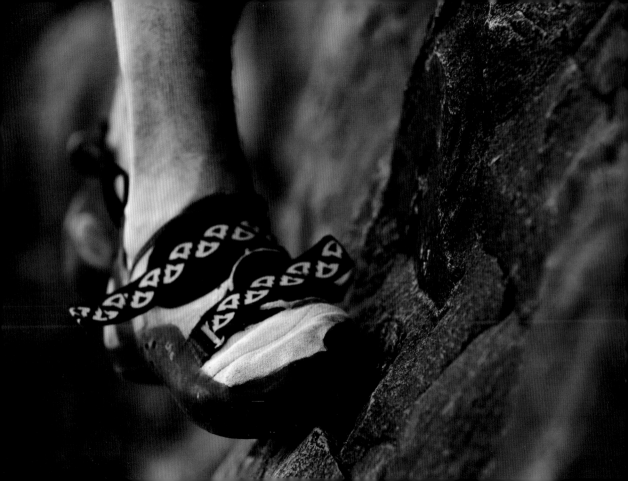

HEATED VERSUS NOT HEATED

Heated yoga rooms are fairly common, particularly in yoga studios. There's a wide variety in approach. Bikram or Hot Hatha practices generally reach temperatures of at least 100 degrees. Most power or vinyasa flow practices, such as the ones you have learned in this book, are taught with some heat, generally in the mid-80s to mid-90s. Unheated classes are taught at room temperature.

The idea behind heat is that it opens your body and helps you sweat to detoxify. Some people love the intense rinse of a heated class. Others prefer to build heat internally through the practice. You may discover you love a big, sweaty practice. Or, you may find you need a balance between the two. Keep in mind some people find their bodies do not tolerate heated practices well.

FLOW

Ashtanga is the original flow practice. Sun Salutation A and B as you have learned in this book are rooted in this style, as is vinyasa flow, or connecting poses with breath. Many teachers credit Ashtanga for teaching them discipline and flow—it is considered an extremely rigorous practice.

Many different types of descriptions of practices will use the word "flow," but they all are likely to rely on a connection of breath and poses moving together. Some focus on one breath per movement through the practice, while other practices allow more time for holding poses, more common in "power yoga" classes. Some types of practices work with a set sequence, such as Ashtanga and Baptiste Power Yoga, while others will sequence to work different areas of the body or build to a particular pose.

HATHA

All yoga is a hatha practice, but these days hatha usually indicates a nonflow practice; the best known of these, Bikram, founded by Bikram Choudhury, features classes held in intense heat. The studios use mirrors for you to focus your gaze, and the Bikram sequence is a set series of twenty-six poses that stays the same regardless of the teacher.

Iyengar, created by yoga master B. K. S. Iyengar, is another nonflow practice that moves from pose to pose, working deeply and precisely into alignment with a focus on healing the body and mind through poses. An Iyengar practice uses many props and fine-tunes alignment with long holds.

KUNDALINI

Kundalini means "serpent power" and is an energetic practice that might include waving your hands or closing and opening your hands over and over. It also includes meditation, poses, mantra, and breathing techniques.

GENTLE OR YIN

Also known as restorative yoga, this style is geared toward restoring your body from intense athletic days, or for people with injuries or other physical challenges who want to breathe and move at a slower, modified pace. A yin practice will take you through long deep holds, while a gentle class could show up as a modified flow practice or moving from pose to pose. If you climb intensely almost every day, consider taking a restorative practice once a week.

STEP 3: IDENTIFY TEACHERS WHO ELEVATE YOU

When a teacher is great, he inspires me to hold a pose longer or take the extra Wheel, especially when I don't want to. If a teacher is great *and* funny, he can make me laugh. I love those classes. When it comes to your yoga practice, a great teacher can be the difference between staying committed and giving up.

The first step to looking for a teacher is looking at her credentials. Make sure she comes from an established yoga training program. In addition to training, experience is a helpful indicator. The more time a teacher has spent understanding the body, how to read a class of different body types and experiences, and how to speak to the body in a way that makes sense to you, the more impact she will have on you and your practice. Most yoga teachers also assist in poses to support your alignment, and a great assist can make the difference between struggle and freedom in a pose.

Beyond that, a great teacher resonates with you personally. You may find you prefer the sequences taught by a particular teacher. You may find you need a funny teacher to get through a challenging class. You may be drawn to a gentle teacher who gives you space to grow, or you may find yourself going back to a teacher who has heart and passion to challenge you to new depth in your poses.

Lastly, find more than one teacher. Every teacher, whether at a community center near your home or at a yoga studio, has something to share. You may be surprised when a teacher you initially didn't like grows on you. Listen and learn along the way, and you will not only find new teachers to support you, you'll learn something about yourself.

STEP 4: CREATE YOUR YOGA COMMUNITY

Like a climbing buddy who encourages you to sport climb on a day you considered staying in bed, a community can help you stick with your yoga practice. As you search for a place to practice, observe the community. Do people chat before and after class? Does the person at the front desk know your name? Does the teacher ask people to introduce themselves to each other?

You may be tempted to isolate yourself in practice, particularly when you are new. But practicing with a teacher also means practicing with other people, and community is a powerful element of yoga. Like the other climbers who became instant friends because you shared the same route, a class full of like-minded people may be just what you need to thrive.

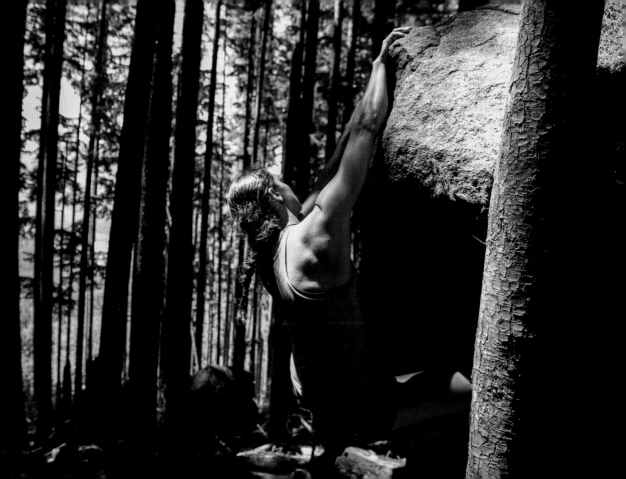

CHAPTER 7
EATING MINDFULLY

WHAT YOU EAT FUELS your body. It's a simple concept, and yet it can feel very complicated when you dive into the world of nutrition. For someone who is active, it matters even more that you get enough calories to sustain yourself through a yoga class or on long days out on the wall.

There is no right way to eat mindfully. But the first step is to notice whether you pay attention to what you eat in the first place.

The world is rife with cleanses, diets, and other challenges. I have tried many of them, some for myself and some in the name of research. I have at times cut out sugar, alcohol, gluten, dairy, grains, legumes, red meat, processed food, caffeine, canola oil, sweetened drinks, and fruit. Thank goodness for vegetables. I've done an anti-inflammatory diet; I've eaten only fruit; I've gone Paleo; I've done a vegan cleanse; I've limited my meals to five times a day with a plate two-thirds full of veggies and fruit.

What's the point of all this cleansing? Every time I've experienced one, I've noticed something about my food habits. Eliminating a certain food or type of food for a short time has helped me recognize when I was eating out of habit and convenience versus choosing the best food for my body. Through my experience, I've found it is best to eat foods in which you recognize all the ingredients. It's even better if you know where it comes from, and it's helpful for the environment if it originates close to home.

But I've also learned that every person's body is different. What works for one person may not work for another.

Every year, I lead a three-day fruit cleanse with yoga students in my "40 Days to Personal Revolution" program. At the meeting leading up to the cleanse, I always hear diverse, creative excuses for why people can't do it. Some are traveling. Others already have dinner planned with friends on all three nights of the cleanse. Some question whether it's healthy to eat so much (natural) sugar for three days.

Ultimately for many students, doing the cleanse is simply a triumph of commitment. Some appreciate discovering how fixated they are on food. Others learn that they are addicted to their morning cup of coffee. One mom realized she snacks constantly while fixing her kids' food for the day, a mindless habit.

The three-day fruit cleanse is one real-life step to bringing your yoga practice to your day-to-day life. You may already have noticed how eating habits impact how you feel during yoga, for example. Having wine the night before an early morning class might make it feel rather challenging. Or you might be in a twist, and with a groan, realize whatever you ate wasn't quite right.

These days, I know my body does best when I eat at home, cooking vegetables, whole grains and humanely raised meat, along with some fruit. I tend to eat seasonally, particularly with fruits and vegetables, and love to shop at my local farmers' market in the summer. If I'm eating out alone, I pick a salad or something healthy, most days. If I'm out with friends or family, I enjoy myself. When I'm headed out to climb, my favorite thing to eat is a sandwich and a brownie from a local bakery. Of all the days to eat whatever I want, a day outside definitely wins.

Still, I like a nutrition challenge every three months or so to put some awareness back on how I've been eating. Sometimes I do a cleanse because I want to lose a couple pounds. Sometimes I do a challenge to balance out energy slumps during the day. Other times, I've been eating out a lot, and I'm ready to bring some more mindfulness to my diet.

In addition to evaluating your food choices, you may want to consider other mindfulness practices that will make you feel healthier. I try to sleep at least seven hours a night, which is simple if not easy; it feels like a healthy amount for me. However when I pay attention to my sleep, I do tend to sleep even more.

Below are a few practices to eating mindfully, two modified from some of my favorite resources on this topic: *Savor*, which delves into both nutrition and mindfulness practices; and *The Abascal Way*. Whatever way you choose to approach mindful eating, know that you can always make a shift simply by paying attention to what you eat!

Apple Meditation Practice

This practice is modified from *Savor: Mindful Eating, Mindful Life* by Thich Nhat Hanh and Dr. Lilian Cheung, which advises, "Eating an apple consciously is to have a new awareness of the apple, of our world, and of our own life."

» Take an apple. Wash it. Before you take a bite, look at it. Take a few deep breaths in and out. Observe the color and the shape. Smell it. What kind of apple is it? Consider the tree where the apple grew, the orchard where the tree lives.

Think about the person who plucked the apple, the people who drove or flew the apple to your city, the people who brought the apple to your grocery store.

» Slowly take a bite. Savor the texture as you bite into the apple. Notice the give of the skin and the crisp flesh underneath. Eat it slowly, taking twenty or so chews to finish your bite. Is it sweet, tart, juicy, or crisp? Notice how the texture changes as you chew. What does it feel like when you swallow?

» Savor the taste of the apple. Chew consciously, savoring the taste, and immersing yourself completely in the apple. Eat the entire apple this way.

Mindful Eating Practice

Bring mindfulness to your diet by eliminating one of the following. Or, if you are feeling bold, choose two or more! Note that both caffeine and sugar are stimulants (caffeine can affect sleep), while alcohol is a depressant. Sugar and alcohol are inflammatory for all people.

Choose to eliminate one or more of these items for one week:

» **Caffeine**: If you drink coffee regularly, replace your morning cup with two cups of green tea for two days before eliminating caffeine entirely.

» **Alcohol**: Abstain from all types of alcohol.

» **Processed foods**: Do not eat any packaged food that includes ingredients you can't identify.

» **Tobacco**: Cut out all tobacco.

» **Sugar**: Refrain from eating foods with added sugar, including all refined sugars and natural sweeteners like honey, agave, maple syrup, and other natural sweeteners. This definition includes soft drinks. Note that many packaged foods use sugar identified by different names, like dextrose, maltose, sucrose, etc.

No Midnight Snacks! Practice

This practice is adapted from "The TQI Diet," described in *The Abascal Way* by Kathy Abascal.

» Stop eating two to three hours before bed.

As adults, we have one daily burst of hormone that occurs a few hours after we fall asleep, which helps maintain muscle mass as we age. But if you eat a bedtime snack, "the insulin released will shut down the important burst of growth hormone that night" writes Abascal.

Eating before bed over time also sends signals to your brain to change your normal hunger and satiety signals. Humans are supposed to be hungry in the morning, not at night. Leptin, the hormone that is tied to satiety also affects melatonin, which is released during the night. If you give up your bedtime snack, people typically notice "they are sleeping better and feel more clearheaded during the day," says Abascal.

LIKE YOGA, EATING MINDFULLY is a practice, and it takes time to shift patterns. Don't take it too seriously if you go off the path on occasion. Remember your intention. Observe what feels best in your body and choose from there.

RESOURCES

BOOKS

Abascal, Kathy. *The Abascal Way: To Quiet Inflammation*. Vashon: Tigana Press, 2011.

Baptiste, Baron. *40 Days to Personal Revolution: A Breakthrough Program to Radically Change Your Body and Awaken the Sacred within Your Soul*. New York: Simon and Schuster, 2004.

———. *Journey into Power: How to Sculpt Your Ideal Body, Free Your True Self, and Transform Your Life with Yoga*. New York: Simon and Schuster, 2002.

Desikachar, T. K. V. *The Heart of Yoga: Developing a Personal Practice*. Rochester, VT: Inner Traditions International, 1999.

Hartranft, Chip and Patañjali. *The Yoga-Sūtra of Patañjali: A New Translation with Commentary*. Boston: Shambhala Publications, 2003.

Iyengar, B. K. S. *Light on Life: The Yoga Journey to Wholeness, Inner Peace, and Ultimate Freedom*. Emmaus, PA: Rodale, 2005.

———. *Light on Yoga*. New York: Schocken Books, 1979.

Kaminoff, Leslie. *Yoga Anatomy*. Champaign, IL: Human Kinetics, 2007.

Long, Ray. *The Key Muscles of Yoga: Your Guide to Functional Anatomy in Yoga*. Bandha Yoga Publications, 2006.

———. *The Key Poses of Yoga: Your Guide to Functional Anatomy in Yoga*. Bandha Yoga Publications, 2008.

Nhat Hanh, Thich, and Lilian Cheung. *Savor: Mindful Eating, Mindful Life*. New York: HarperOne, 2010.

MAGAZINES AND OTHER RESOURCES

Chopra Center for Wellbeing, www.chopra.com: Meditation resource

Yoga Alliance, www.yogaalliance.org: National yoga teacher directory

Yoga Journal, www.yogajournal.com: Leading national yoga magazine and website

INDEX

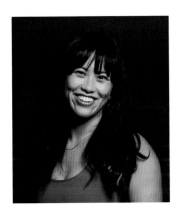

Nicole Tsong writes the popular "Fit for Life" column in the *Seattle Times*, published in *Pacific NW Magazine*. Tsong teaches yoga at Seattle's leading yoga studios, where she runs strong, essential, and fun classes, leads retreats, and trains and mentors new yoga teachers. She is a Certified Baptiste Teacher and a leader in the national yoga community. Tsong is a member of the board for Seattle-based nonprofit Yoga Behind Bars. She now lives in Seattle. Formerly an award-winning reporter for the *Seattle Times* and the *Anchorage Daily News*, she has traveled to Nome, Alaska, to cover the finish line of the world-renowned Iditarod dog-sled race and covered politics in Washington, DC.

Erika Schultz shares stories through documentary photography and video. A staff photographer for the *Seattle Times*, she was raised in central Wyoming and attended college at Northern Arizona University and Syracuse University in London. She is a cofounder of NW Photojournalism and an SPJ Western Washington board member.

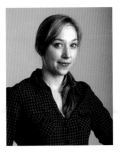

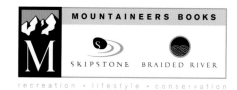
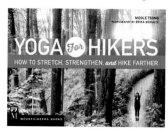
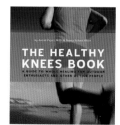
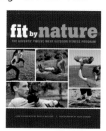